A DOCTOR'S ANSWER TO

TENNIS ELBOW

HOW TO CURE IT
HOW TO PREVENT IT

Beckett Howorth, M.D.
& Fred Bender

CHELSEA HOUSE
New York, London
1977

Project Editor: **Ingrid Russell**
Art Director: **Susan Lusk**
Managing Editor: **Laurie Likoff**
Illustrator: **Tony Malone**

Library of Congress Cataloging in Publication Data
Howorth, M Beckett, 1902-
A doctor's answer to tennis elbow.

1. Tennis elbow. 2. Tennis—Physiological aspects. I. Bender, Fred, 1923- joint author. II. Title. RD558.H68 617'.17 77-4145 ISBN 0-87754-052-7

CHELSEA HOUSE PUBLISHERS

Harold Steinberg, Chairman & Publisher   Andrew E. Norman, President
A Division of Chelsea House Educational Communications, Inc.
70 West 40th Street. New York, N.Y. 10018

A DOCTOR'S ANSWER TO TENNIS ELBOW
HOW TO CURE IT
HOW TO PREVENT IT

TABLE OF CONTENTS

PREFACE

Tennis elbow. What is it? What causes it? How is it treated? How can it be prevented?

As an orthopedist, I have been asked these questions by hundreds of patients with this injury. Their number increases as interest in the sport grows. In fact, tennis elbow is one of the most frequent complaints I now treat. The problem is almost epidemic, frustrating and incapacitating an estimated ten to fifteen million players in the United States. In addition, the mere possibility of having tennis elbow makes many more players apprehensive. The methods of prevention and cure run the gamut from magic beads to surgery.

Because the problem is so widespread and because authoritative information about it is so needed, I joined with my coauthor, a consultant in the health field and a knowledgeable tennis player, to write this book. Our purpose is to separate fact from fiction and to provide a comprehensive guide to the prevention and cure of the tennis elbow injury.

Tennis players, like all athletes, are vulnerable to strains and injuries. If you are a weekend player, you may be more vulnerable than the everyday player. It all depends on your physical condition, and on whether you follow a routine conditioning and warm-up program, stroke correctly, and use the proper equipment. By following the techniques outlined in this book, you will become less vulnerable, not only to tennis elbow but to other tennis-related injuries. Our emphasis, however, will be on tennis elbow since it is the most common and debilitating problem.

The term "tennis elbow" refers to a group of injuries which occur in the elbow area, caused by many activities besides tennis. Any ball or racket game can cause or aggravate it, as can such diverse activities as raking leaves, using a screwdriver, twisting open a jar cap, or simply banging the outer elbow. One of the prime causes, of course, is repeatedly hitting a tennis ball with an incorrect stroke. But any abrupt movement of the elbow, especially if it is done with force or against resistance, can initiate an attack. No matter what the cause, the symptoms are similar: a persistent soreness in the elbow area ranging from mildly annoying to severely painful. And, as you will see, the basic curative and preventive measures are the same.

Hopefully, you don't have tennis elbow and are reading this book because you're interested in preventing it. But perhaps you already have it. Your attack may be mild and transient, or it may be severe and persistent. If you have a continuing or recurring problem, this book should be of special importance to you. By following the simple programs described, you'll find that you **can** eliminate the discomfort and pain in your elbow. And because our therapy program will help you recondition your arm and restore its vitality, you should no longer have recurrent attacks. You will be able to play again without pain, without apprehension, and without apologies.

PRELIMINARIES

ONE
A CASE HISTORY

While planning this book, I asked a typical patient to write about his tennis elbow experience as accurately as he could. The patient is forty-two years old, has a sedentary job and recently developed a passion for tennis. His words are worth quoting in their entirety:

"All my adult life I have felt a need for a regimen of exercise—some sort of physical activity to maintain a sense of well-being and fitness. I have bowled, golfed, swum, jogged, lifted weights, biked, done yoga and Canadian Air Force exercises and tried a number of other activities that usually lasted from a week to several months.

"Two years ago a friend invited me to join him on the tennis court. Until then I had never held a tennis racket in my hand, and my only knowledge of the game was that one attempts to hit the ball over the net so that the opponent can't return it—same as ping-pong, so I thought. I was shown how to hold the racket, given a few minutes of instruction on how to hit the ball, and we started to play tennis. To my amazement and chagrin I could not return the ball in court: I either missed it entirely or hit it feebly into the net or forceably over the fence. It was a very disappointing afternoon. I felt inept, clumsy, and frustrated; but I was determined to learn to play.

"I read several tennis instruction books, watched a few

professional tennis games, practiced hitting the ball against a wall and played whenever I got a chance. I gradually began to control hitting the ball over the net and into the court. During the learning process, I developed an affection for the game that I had never experienced with any other sport or exercise. I played for several months, and the more I played the better I became. I was delighted that at last I had found a sport I enjoyed and wanted to continue. Although I was aware of a slight pain in my forearm each time I played, I didn't give it too much thought. In fact, that summer I was already planning my winter vacation around the idea of playing tennis in some warm climate. Then it happened.

"I was awakened at 4 a.m. It was an alarm from my aching forearm and not my clock. I was disturbed by the throbbing pain, but since I had played tennis for several hours the day before I simply thought that I had overdone it. I decided to take it easy for a day or two and cancel my tennis appointments for the weekend. I had had similar aches in the past, in the thigh, shoulder, back, and neck, but they all had disappeared after a few days of adequate rest. However, unlike these other pains, the one in my forearm did not go away. For the next few days I rested my arm except for washing, getting dressed, brushing my teeth, and turning the ignition key—all relatively easy movements which became more and more painful.

"Within a week I started switching ordinary right-hand movements to my left hand, occasionally shaking hands absentmindedly with my right. These moments of forgetfulness caused extreme pain in my forearm and elbow. Since the most acute pain seemed to be centered in the elbow, it was not difficult for me to guess that I had tennis elbow. After seven days and nights of pain and restricted right-hand-and-arm movements, I found no relief. I was distraught and went to my family doctor.

"He confirmed my diagnosis: I was indeed a victim of tennis elbow. Although no swelling was visible, I had somehow caused an injury to the structure in and around the elbow joint. I was advised to rest my arm, preferably in a sling, and was told not to lift so much as a postage stamp. I was given a prescription for an anti-inflammatory pill and sent home—'not to worry, a very common ailment these days, many patients complain of the same thing.' The anti-inflammatory pills caused dizziness and disturbed vision, and I was advised to stop taking them. Since my elbow still ached, I was told to take aspirin instead of the prescription pills. Two weeks of aspirin and still no relief—and no tennis. My symptoms: couldn't fully extend my arm or lift a coffee cup or brush my teeth without discomfort. Not being able to play tennis was one thing, but being elbowed out of the mere performance of daily functions was another!

"I talked to other tennis elbow sufferers and they told me to see a particular orthopedist, a specialist in sports-related injuries. After a careful examination and many questions about my game, the specialist confirmed that I had tennis elbow and gave me a shot of cortisone. As the needle went into my elbow, the pain was momentarily stunning. However, within an hour the pain subsided and all the symptoms of tennis elbow vanished.

"The orthopedist cautioned me about the possibility of getting tennis elbow again. He handed me a gripping device and told me to squeeze it as hard as I could. The dial on the contraption registered the strength of my gripping prowess. To my surprise and near shame, my score was below average and what's more, according to the doctor, I had a set of underconditioned muscles in my forearm. Therefore, I was particularly vulnerable to a recurrence of tennis elbow in the future. To strengthen my muscle tone, the doctor taught me a series of hand and arm exercises that would build more power in my grip, wrist, and forearm before I resumed the rigors of tennis. In addition, he suggested that I review my strokes with a tennis instructor to make sure that I wasn't abusing my arm.

"I started the exercises several days after my visit. As the doctor had predicted, the pain was gone completely and I began to feel as good as new. Within a week, I was back on the court. I forgot my previous pain—and the strengthening exercises as well. Within a month, the pain in my elbow had returned with a vengeance. Yes, I had been forewarned. Had I consistently followed the doctor's program for gradual rehabilitation, I might have been out on the court that very afternoon, working up a sweat, trying for new victories and having the time of my life. Instead, there I was—standing, I should say, cowering, in front of my doctor while he readied the hypodermic for another cortisone shot.

"As the needle entered my elbow, I secretly swore off tennis forever. The pain disappeared as before. This time, not only did I start the exercise program, but I have continued it conscientiously every day. Months have passed since my last treatment. Occasionally I feel a slight twinge of pain when I lift a heavy object at some particular angle, but these incidents are rare. I now use my arm normally without discomfort. The other day, while cleaning out a closet, I came across my racket. It felt good to pick it up and swing it against the air. Someday soon I think I'll be ready to try it again with a ball and net."

This patient has not returned to my office since his last treatment, but his tale does not end there. I called him several weeks ago to see how he was doing. I was not surprised to learn that he was playing tennis again three or four times a week. He told me he had attended a tennis clinic where his strokes were analyzed and corrected. He had had no further problems with his elbow and attributed this to the improvement in his strokes and to his faithful following of the exercises that you will find in "Preventive Conditioning" (chapter 9).

TWO
VULNERABILITY TEST

Before getting into a more complete discussion of the tennis elbow injury, let's find out just how vulnerable you are to getting it.

After questioning, examining, and treating hundreds of tennis elbow patients, I find that they share certain characteristics that can be readily pin-pointed. If you were to consult a sports-injury-oriented orthopedist, you probably would be asked some of the following questions. Your answers would help the doctor determine what caused the injury, how to treat it, and how to help you prevent its recurrence.

The Vulnerability Test that follows will help you decide if you are a likely candidate for tennis elbow or, if you already have it, what might have caused it. To rate your vulnerability, answer each question as best you can before reading on.

	YES	NO	SOMEWHAT or SOMETIMES	
1.	____	____	____	Do you often have difficulty twisting open jar lids?
2.	____	____	____	When you shake hands, does the other person's handshake always seem stronger than yours?
3.	____	____	____	Do you have difficulty crushing empty soda or beer cans with one hand?

	YES	NO	SOMEWHAT or SOMETIMES	
4.	____	____	____	When playing tennis does your grip often tire or slip?
5.	____	____	____	Would you describe your forearm muscles as underdeveloped?
6.	____	____	____	Are your upper arm muscles flabby?
7.	____	____	____	Does your arm tire easily when you are carrying a shopping bag or suitcase?
8.	____	____	____	After half an hour of play, does your tennis racket feel heavier than when you started?
9.	____	____	____	Do you maintain a regular exercise program?
10.	____	____	____	Do you consider yourself in good physical condition?
11.	____	____	____	Do you warm up regularly before playing a game?
12.	____	____	____	If you warm up, do you do so for more than ten minutes?
13.	____	____	____	Do you stop playing when you are overtired?
14.	____	____	____	Did you pay attention to grip size, weight, stringing, and flexibility when selecting your racket?
15.	____	____	____	Did you learn to play with little or no instruction?
16.	____	____	____	Do you consider your strokes unorthodox or have you been told that they are?
17.	____	____	____	Do you often hit the ball off-center?

	YES	NO	SOMEWHAT or SOMETIMES	
18.	____	____	____	Do you find it difficult to keep your eye on the ball while playing?
19.	____	____	____	Do you often run around your backhand?
20.	____	____	____	Do you often try for power in your strokes?

Your answers to these 20 questions cannot reveal with certainty whether you will be a victim of tennis elbow or not. However, they can serve as a good guide to your vulnerability and can indicate where your strengths and weaknesses lie.

Questions 1 through 8 relate to the strength and development of the muscles in your arm, wrist, and hand. If you answered all or a majority of the questions

NO: Low Vulnerability You probably have strong hand and arm muscles. Continue spot exercises for the maintenance and development of your muscle tone.

SOMEWHAT/SOMETIMES: Moderate Vulnerability Your hand and arm muscles require strengthening: do not neglect following a program of spot exercises.

YES: High Vulnerability You are in a danger area, risking injury to your elbow. You should adopt a conscientious program of developing the muscles of your hand, wrist, forearm, and upper arm.

Questions 9 through 14 relate to your overall physical fitness and condition, and your knowledge of the selection of proper tennis equipment. If you answered all or a majority of the questions

YES: Low Vulnerability You are probably in good physical condition. Continue your exercise program of physical fitness. Jogging or running a mile or more four to six times a week will build your stamina for the tennis court.

SOMEWHAT/SOMETIMES: Moderate Vulnerability You

require a more disciplined and regular exercise program for the improvement of your physical fitness and endurance.
NO: High Vulnerability You are a prime target for tennis elbow and other injuries that can be sustained while playing. Tennis requires agility, strength, endurance and coordination. It is important for you to start a program to improve your general physical capacity.

Questions 15 through 20 relate to your basic tennis techniques. If you answered all or a majority of the questions
NO: Low Vulnerability You are well trained for tennis. Continue practice drills for the improvement of weak areas.
SOMEWHAT/SOMETIMES: Moderate Vulnerability You should spend more time developing stroke technique through practice drills. Joining a tennis clinic or class can be especially helpful in correcting poor habits formed over a period of time.
YES: High Vulnerability There are no shortcuts to learning how to play tennis properly. Attention to basic strokes, footwork, and body movements are all essential requirements of the game. Proper instruction and continued practice will help you overcome your tennis-playing difficulties.

No matter how you've scored on the Vulnerability Test, you will have a better understanding of tennis elbow if, as you read through the next chapter, you examine your own arm or that of a friend.

THREE
HOW YOUR ARM WORKS

The aching elbow has plagued man throughout the ages whenever he overburdened the muscle-tendon-ligament structure of his arm. The syndrome of tennis elbow was first described in a medical journal in 1873, the same year that tennis was introduced in Wales as a new game. Since that time, whenever a carpenter, painter, gardener, or luggage porter injured his elbow while performing his job, the injury has been referred to as "tennis elbow." It is tennis players, however, who are most often affected with this malady.

This chapter takes a quick look at the basic structure of the arm, how it functions, and how it relates to tennis elbow. With the aid of the diagrams, you'll be able to distinguish the various components of the arm and see how they function in the tennis stroke. This should help you understand how the elbow gets injured and, consequently, what you can do to avoid this injury. If you are already suffering from tennis elbow, it should help your understanding of the rehabilitation process.

Three bones form the basic skeletal structure of the arm: the humerus, the radius, and the ulna. Muscles, which move these bones, are attached to them either directly or by means of tendons. Since bones are almost rigid, motion occurs only at the joints where bones meet: these contact areas, called articulations, are constructed to permit specific movements. Ligaments of connective tissue hold the bones together at the joints in such a way as to allow these movements. The ligaments form capsules, enclosing the joints, whose membranes secrete a lubricating fluid which smooths the interaction of the articulations. The elbow is a joint at which the three bones of the arm converge with several areas of contact. However, it is not only your elbow articulations and forearm and wrist muscles which are active in tennis stroking. Your shoulder joints and muscles of the upper arm participate as well.

In the upper arm there is only one bone, the humerus, which extends from shoulder to elbow. At the upper end of the humerus is a rounded head that fits into a cavity at the outer side of the shoulder blade. This fitting, forming a ball-and-socket joint, allows great mobility of the arm so that we can swing it around like a windmill and in many directions. Also at the upper end of the humerus, but on the outer side, there's a knob (the greater tuberosity) to which muscles are anchored, controlling certain motions of the shoulder pertinent to the tennis stroke. You can feel the head and the tuberosity under the muscles if you roll your shoulder under your finger and thumb. The shoulder contributes much to the power of the tennis stroke if the stroke is executed correctly (see chapter 8).

The shaft of the humerus is long and slender and widens at the elbow, where you can easily feel two distinct knobs, one on each side. The smaller knob on the outer side of the elbow is the lateral epicondyle, while the larger knob on the inner side of the elbow is the medial epicondyle. The lateral epicondyle area is more frequently injured by tennis players. The injury, medically referred to as "epicondylitis," is commonly called "tennis elbow."

In the forearm, the ulna and the radius extend from elbow to wrist. To feel the ulna, start at the knob just above your wrist on the little finger side, and trace up to and behind the elbow where there is another knob, the olecranon. In front of the olecranon there's a hidden hollow where part of the lower end of the humerus fits, forming a hinge joint. Unlike the ball-and-socket joint at the shoulder, this articula-

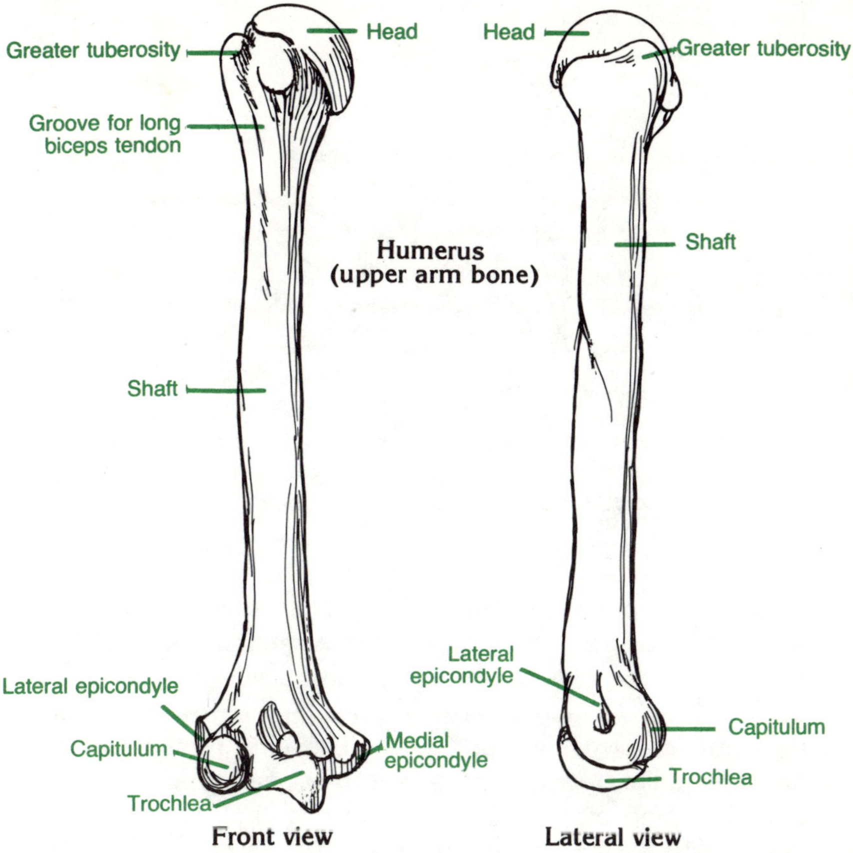

tion is similar to the knee joint, in that it can only move back and forth like a hinged door. This movement is called flexion (toward the shoulder) and extension.

The radius is much more difficult to feel through the skin because it is partly covered by a pad of muscle. Starting at the prominence slightly above your wrist on the thumb side, you can trace the radius upward toward your elbow. The bone can be felt about halfway up the forearm; then it disappears under the muscle, surfacing again at the elbow on the lateral epicondyle side. At the elbow joint is the head of the radius, the upper end of which is saucer-shaped and neatly fits against a knob of the humerus, the capitulum (little head). There is an additional articulation between the head of the radius and a small hidden concavity on the outer side of the ulna in which the radial head revolves, enabling you to turn your palm down, called **"pro-**

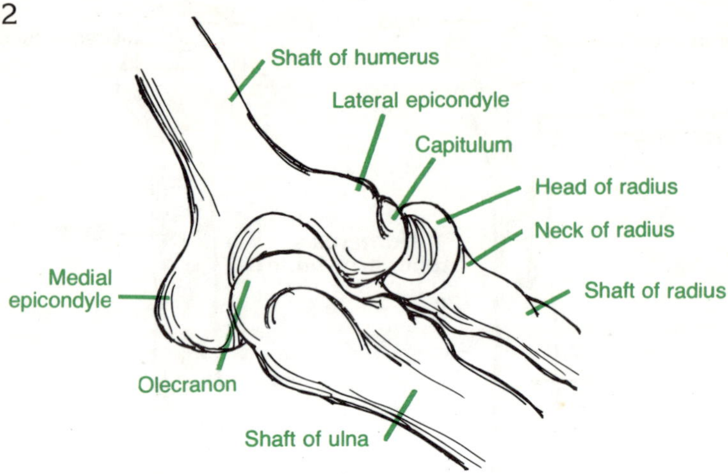

Skeletal components of the elbow

nation," or up, called **"supination."** The radio-humeral joint allows the forearm to be flexed and extended. You can feel the head of the radius moving on the outside of your elbow by cupping your fingers around your bent elbow and rotating your forearm back and forth. The ulna remains stable and the radius revolves around it in pronation and supination. Repeated pronation with the forehand stroke and supination with the backhand are major factors in tennis elbow. (Further along in our muscle explanation, we shall see why this is so; and for more details, see chapter 8.)

The muscles of the arm are numerous; we are not going to describe them all. However, we will indicate the main groups that are important in tennis stroking, and how their weakness or injury can result in tennis elbow. As we mentioned earlier, muscles are attached to the bones, either directly or by means of tendons, which are tough fibrous cords. When a muscle or tendon undergoes excessive stretching, the resulting injury is a **strain** which is usually accompanied by slight swelling and local tenderness. The words tendon and ligament are often used interchangeably but, despite their similar composition, their functions are not the same. As we have seen, ligaments are tough fibrous bands of connective tissue that bind joints together yet allow their specific motions. (Connective tissue is variable in struc-

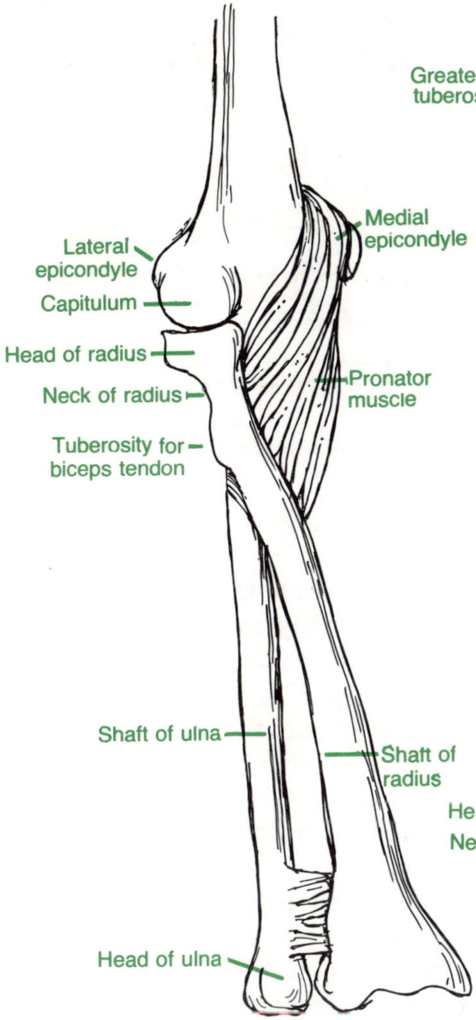

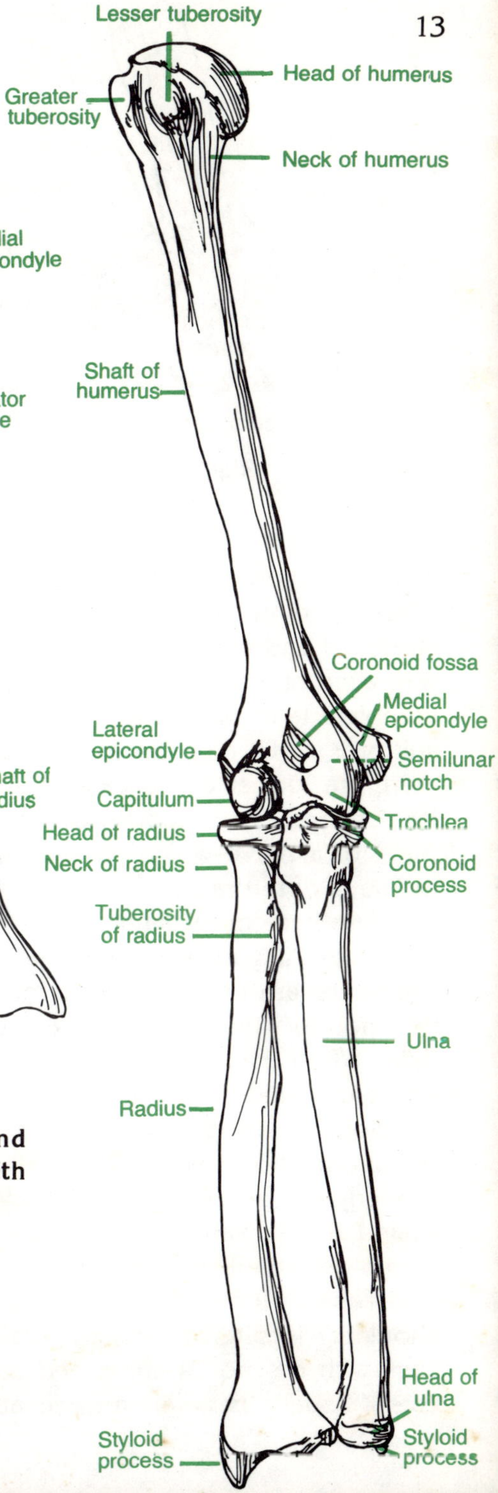

Bones of the arm and forearm, shown above with radius in pronation

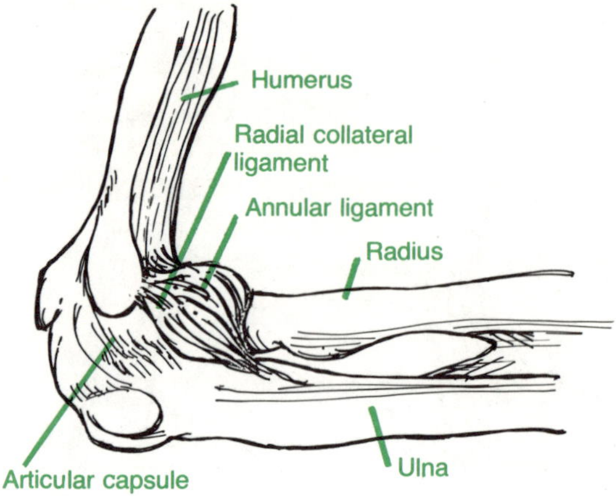

Right elbow joint showing ligaments

ture; it is white, strong, and inelastic, as you may notice the next time you carve a chicken or cut a piece of meat.) When extreme force is exerted on a ligament, it is overstretched and can tear, resulting in an injury called a **sprain**, with accompanying pain and swelling. Sometimes there is a complete tear, or rupture. Tennis elbow is commonly a result of a strain, a sprain or a rupture. (However, occasionally there are further complications such as injury to the articular cartilage of the radial head or the capitulum, or entrapment of a nerve which passes through muscles in front of the neck of the radius.)

Another complication concerns the capsules enclosing the joints. As you may recall, these capsules, formed by the ligaments, are lined with a membrane (similar to that inside the mouth) which normally secretes a lubricating (synovial) fluid. When there has been trauma (injury) to the arm and elbow this fluid production and absorption process can malfunction, resulting in more difficult joint movement and a stiffer and more painful elbow. However, when we exercise properly the production and absorption rates are increased, easing things again. This is why "Exercises for Recovery" are so important (see chapter 6).

Tennis elbow (as well as a similar tendon injury in the shoulder) is often mistakenly called bursitis. A bursa is a sack with a synovial lining and a little fluid, strategically located, usually between muscle and bone, to diminish friction. Occasionally, with a shoulder injury the bursa may be involved secondarily. However, in both locations the primary injury is to the tendon and the proper word is tendinitis.

Muscles are arranged in groups, one group balancing another. Usually, when one group contracts the other relaxes. The muscles of the upper arm are divided into two main groups, the flexors and the extensors. Flexion takes place when you bend your arm at the elbow as when raising your hand toward your shoulder. Extension of the arm takes place whenever you straighten your elbow. If these upper arm flexors and extensors are weak, a greater strain is placed on the other forearm muscles and on the joint, thus increasing vulnerability to tennis elbow.

The most important of the flexor group (and probably the best known of all muscles) is the biceps; it is the major muscle of the three that flex the elbow. It arises from the shoulder, passes down the front of the humerus and is attached by its tendon to the upper end of the radius on the inner side just below the elbow. Some people like to contract their biceps to show how strong they are.

The triceps is the extensor muscle of the elbow. It lies at the back of the humerus; it is not used as much as the biceps in daily life and, consequently, it is less developed. The triceps attaches to the olecranon, where it can be felt as a flat ribbon when your arm is extended against resistance.

The muscles of the forearm which control the movements of the wrist, hand, and fingers are arranged in four groups: the flexors, extensors, pronators, and supinators. These muscle groups are directly related to the problem of tennis elbow.

The flexor muscles in the forearm flex the wrist and fingers and are used to grip or to make a fist. They arise from the medial epicondyle, also from the ulna and radius, and then pass downward to be attached by tendons to the wrist and fingers. The extensor muscles, originating at the lateral epicondyle, follow a similar path down to the wrist and fingers; they open the hand and extend the wrist.

Tennis strokes, especially the backhand and serve, require strong and well-developed extensor muscles. However, the extensor muscles in the forearm, like those in the upper arm, are usually not as well developed as the flexors. Everyday activities, such as lifting, contribute to the development of the stronger flexor muscles, whereas there is little daily activity for the extensors. If the weak extensors become overburdened and tend to ache after a game, it's an early indication of vulnerability to tennis elbow.

When you stretch and extend your arm for a wide ball, or stroke incorrectly with a fully extended arm, the extensor muscles and their tendon attachments are at near-maximum tension and therefore most vulnerable to injury. Any added wrist action further tugs at the muscles and tendon attachments. To these traumatic factors, add the vibrations from the impact of the ball, especially with off-center hits and possibly an ill-chosen racket, and the result is excessive strain on the forearm extensor muscles. The strain travels up the extensors to the tendon attachments at the lateral epicondyle where the damage takes place. This is the most common form of tennis elbow.

The medial epicondyle area is not injured as frequently by tennis players, since the action of the tennis stroke does not involve the flexors as often, nor in a manner which places as much strain on them as on the extensors and their tendons. However, I have seen patients who suffer from pain in both the lateral and medial epicondylar areas. Such a patient usually has underdeveloped flexors as well as extensors and often tends to clutch the racket handle continually, thus fatiguing the already weak flexor muscles and their tendons.

In addition, even experienced tennis players with excellent technique and well-developed muscles sometimes fall victim to tennis elbow. Their injury is often located at the medial epicondyle and is commonly caused by hyperpronating the forearm on the serve follow-through. In this action, a player tries to slice the ball with power, twisting his forearm as he follows through on the same side of the body, instead

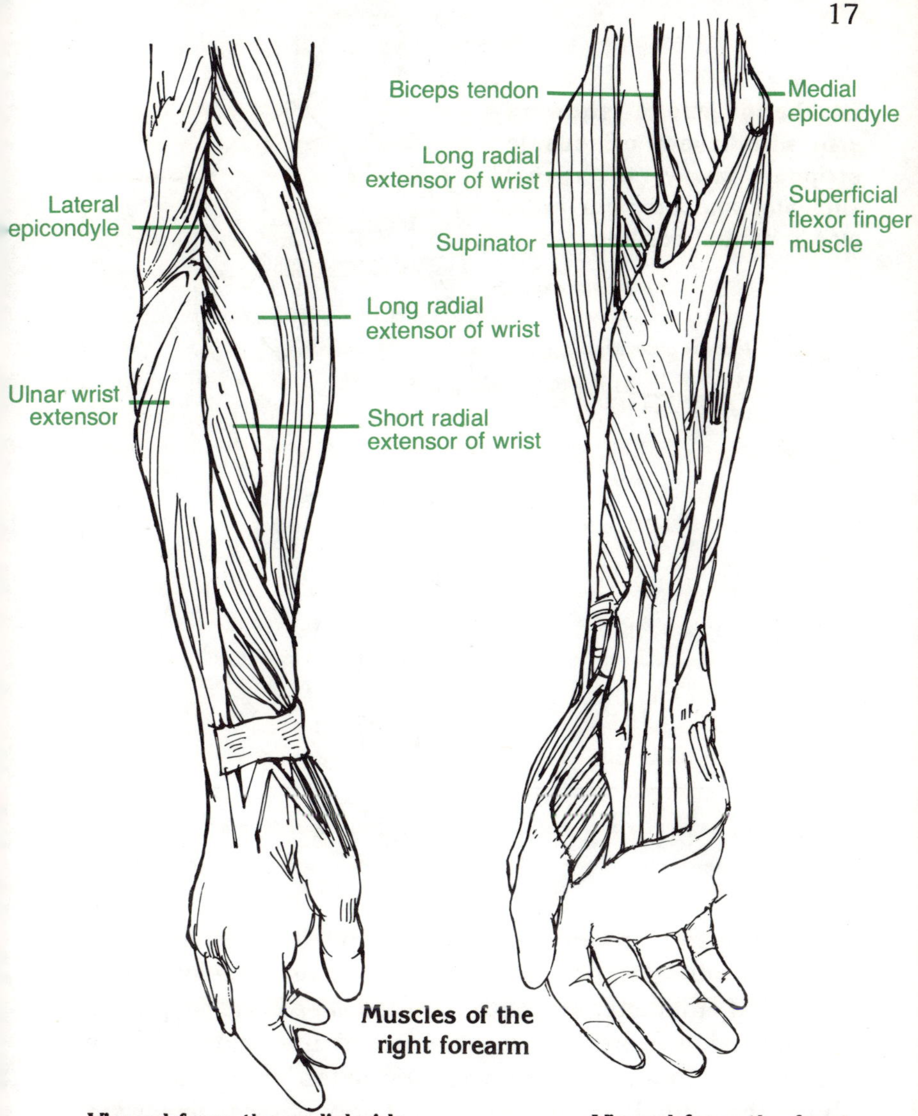

Muscles of the right forearm

Viewed from the radial side **Viewed from the front**

of the opposite side. This exaggerated twisting motion, repeated over and over during serve practice, and combined with the body power behind a strong serve, causes great strain to the medial epicondyle area.

As we mentioned earlier, the terms pronation and supination refer to movements of rotating the forearm palm

Forehand stroke showing arm with layers of muscle stripped away to reveal supinator and pronator muscles in neutral position

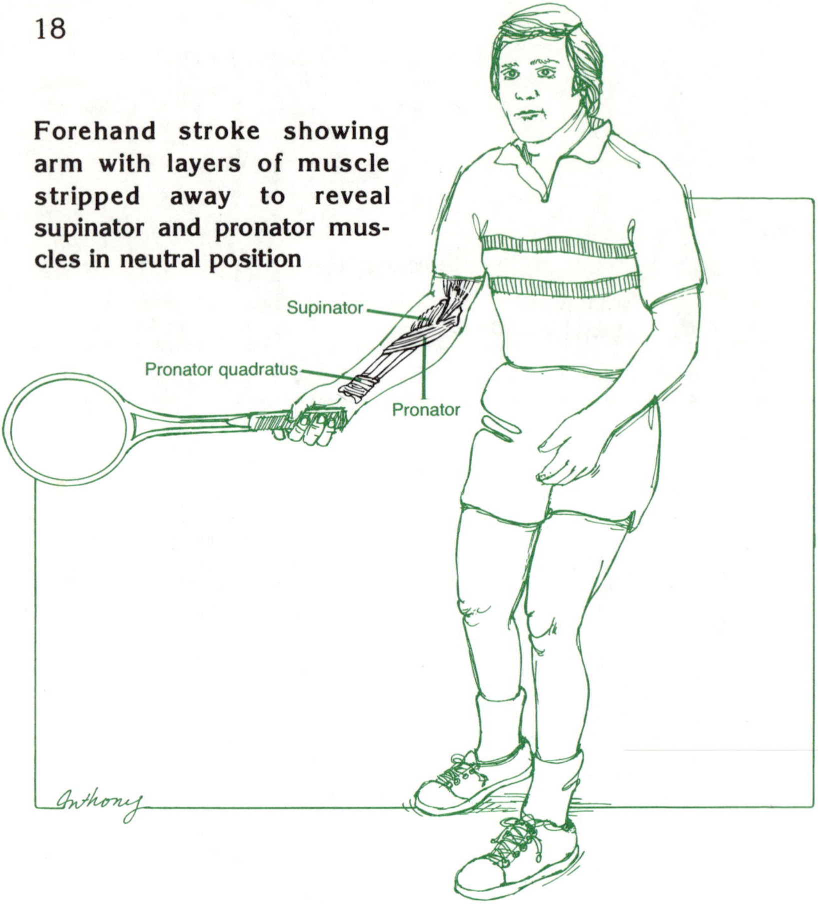

downward and upward respectively, and the pronator and supinator muscles perform these functions. The pronator, beginning at its attachment to the medial epicondyle, passes obliquely downward and is attached to the middle of the radius. The supinator muscle originates at a ridge just above the lateral epicondyle, and it too passes downward and attaches to the radius. Tennis players who stroke with stiff elbows also tend to rotate their forearms on the follow-through. Those who exaggerate pronation and supination incorrectly believe that this is the way to place a spin on the ball. (See "Correct Stroking," chapter 8.) These repeated pronation and supination actions cause tennis elbow by stretching the muscles which consequently overpull their tendons attached to the epicondyles.

Characteristically, tennis elbow is associated with discomfort or pain at or near the epicondyles, but the pain may also extend into the flexor, extensor, pronator, and supinator muscles of the forearm. It is aggravated by jerky movements or by stretching or tightening or contracting the involved muscles. Shaking hands, for instance, tightens the extensor muscles as you reach out, while grasping the offered hand contracts the flexor muscles. And, since the twisting and pumping motion of a handshake pulls on the pronator and supinator muscles, you should avoid shaking hands if you are suffering from tennis elbow. Other activities that use the forearm muscles and their attachments also should be avoided. If you have tennis elbow, turn to the next chapter and you will learn about these "don'ts," as well as about what you can do to help your elbow.

HOW TO CURE IT

FOUR
HOME TREATMENT

From time to time we all experience varying degress of pain. Our general experience with pain has conditioned most of us to believe that it will go away. Unfortunately for the tennis player, the pain in the elbow doesn't usually disappear; and, if it isn't attended to, the pain can worsen.

Pain is a signal sent by our nerves that something has gone wrong and is begging for attention. As we have seen in the previous chapter, the pain of tennis elbow is a result of strain or trauma to the arm muscles, the tendons, the ligaments, the articular cartilage or a combination of these. The strain causes damage, inflammation, stretching or tearing of tissue, or a complete rupture of tissue from its mooring. Usually the pain is located in the forearm muscle and/or on the outer side of the elbow (lateral epicondyle). Tennis elbow is localized, and does not spread to other parts of the body. However, both sides of your elbow may be injured and, if you abuse your other arm, it too may get injured. Occasionally, the elbow is affected by arthritis, or gout, which may coexist with tennis elbow.

There is no direct way of measuring pain or of comparing the pain of different people. Some people tolerate pain better than others; some minimize or ignore it. How bad is your pain? Can you score it from 1 to 10? If your pain is severe, scoring 6 to 10, don't delay seeing your doctor or an orthopedist. If it is mild, scoring 1 to 5, you may still wish to consult your physician nonetheless, for a prolonged injury left unattended is more difficult to treat. Here are seven basic suggestions for home treatment.

1. BE GOOD TO YOUR ARM

"Playing it out" or the "grin and bear it" policy aggravates the pain, increases the inflammation, and prolongs recovery. No matter what your pain is, the first rule is DON'T FURTHER INJURE THE AREA THAT HURTS. Don't do anything that causes pain, such as repeatedly testing the area to see if the pain has suddenly gone. Stay out of the pain zone! If your score is 1 to 5, you may decide to try home-treatment methods of relieving and eliminating the pain. Nature's way of healing an inflammation is rest. Often Nature does quite well. Whenever possible, your hand, arm, and elbow should be at rest when you are not exercising (see "Exercises for Recovery," chapter 6).

2. THE SLING

Allowing your arm to hang at your side can aggravate the pain. A sling, worn part time, can be very helpful. A full triangular sling, with the elbow bent at a right angle is advisable. The narrow cravat sling is not suitable, as it allows the wrist and hand to dangle.

Slings are available at most pharmacies, but one can easily be made at home. To make a sling for the average adult you will need a 42″ square of strong cotton or similar fabric (an old sheet will do). Cut or fold the square in half diagonally or on the bias. To wear the sling, cradle your elbow in the sling corner or right angle, letting the sling extend slightly beyond the elbow. With the sling around your forearm, tie the ends around your neck so that the knot is as comfortable as possible, or use a safety pin. Adjust the sling so that it reaches your knuckles, then have someone help you fold and pin it securely around your elbow. In this way your hand and wrist will be properly supported; if the hand is allowed to dangle, there is a drag on the very muscle you are trying to protect.

Wear the sling as much as you can for as long as it is helpful. If you toss and turn at night, wear it while sleeping. Of course, you may remove it for washing or other personal needs and for doing the exercises in "Exercises for Recovery." If it is impossible to wear the sling during the day because it interferes with your work, try to support your arm whenever possible by slipping your hand into your jacket or shirt, Napoleon-style, hooking your thumb around your belt, or resting your forearm on a table or desk.

3. DON'TS

Of course, don't bang your elbow against anything. (When wearing a sling you may misjudge the distance from elbow to object.) If you tend to do this, you can protect your elbow further by padding it with a piece of foam rubber or a knee pad, generally available in sports shops. Avoid using a screwdriver, hammer, saw, rake, or broom. Don't attempt to open tight lids on bottles and jars. Twisting and turning your hand, wrist and forearm tugs the muscles and tendons, and may increase the injury and evoke pain. Avoid carrying objects suitcase-style, arm stretched and extended at your side. Don't repeatedly grasp and pull as in weeding. Avoid entering the pain zone, even if it means shaking hands with the other hand or bowing from the waist instead. At parties or other functions where such handshaking is required, you might wear a sling for self-protection. Don't overload your healthy arm and hand with duties normally done by your injured arm. If your sore arm was poorly developed before you started playing tennis, it is very likely that your other arm is also poorly developed and is susceptible to tennis elbow. Don't let your arm become chilled while sleeping; avoid drafts from an open window, fan, or air-conditioner. When you go to bed, you can wear a sleeve cut from an old warm sweater. The warmth is comforting, and will promote healing and prevent stiffness in the morning. Don't sleep on your sore arm. One way to protect your arm during sleep is to place it in a sling across your chest and button your pajama top over it to keep it in place. An alternate method would be to secure the "slinged" arm to your body with several turns of an ace bandage encircling your arm and body.

4. MEDICATION

Aspirin is the simplest, safest, and one of the most effective medicines for pain relief. Not only does aspirin diminish pain, it has an anti-inflammatory action as well. The usual adult dose is 2 or 3 tablets, 3 or 4 times daily. You can take aspirin when required, but for no longer than ten days. If there is no relief in that time, you would be well advised to see an orthopedist. In any case, discontinue use if aspirin makes you feel ill. Aspirin sometimes causes slight bleeding in the stomach; it's a good idea to take it after you have eaten rather than when your stomach is empty. At bedtime you can take it with half a glass of milk, an apple, a slice of bread, or an antacid. "Buffered" aspirin is less likely to irritate your stomach. However, if you have or have had a stomach ulcer, you should not take aspirin at all. Various mixtures of other drugs with aspirin are usually more expensive and have little or no added benefit. If you are taking other medications, check with your doctor before you start taking aspirin; a combination of drugs can cause an adverse reaction.

5. COLD

The application of cold is usually more comforting than heat for tennis elbow. Cold is especially useful immediately after a sprain or if a small swelling appears at the elbow, since it tends to shrink swollen or inflamed tissues and acts as a sort of local anesthetic, relieving pain and stiffness. You can apply cold to your elbow by means of cold towels, an ice bag, an alcohol pack, or submersion in a basin of cold water. When you apply any of these methods, your arm should be in a comfortable and supported position. You may use cold for 15 to 20 minutes at a time, several times a day, but for no longer than three days. **A cautionary note:**

Cold can "burn" your skin if it is too cold, or if you use it for too long a time. Naturally, if it causes you any additional pain or discomfort, you should discontinue using it.

6. HEAT

When properly applied, heat stimulates the blood circulation; it is soothing and relaxing and can relieve pain. It's especially useful for mild cases of tennis elbow, when there is a strain and the arm muscles are sore and fatigued from too much activity. You can apply wet or dry heat to your arm or elbow. Whatever method you use, your arm should be in a comfortable and supported position during the treatment. Wet heat can be applied by soaking the arm and elbow in a basin of warm water, at a temperature not exceeding 110° F. Alternatively, a warm towel, wrung out, covered with a thin plastic wrap to retain the heat and prevent dripping, can be used. Dry heat may be applied in a variety of ways: water bag, electric pad, or heat lamp. While using any electric appliance, you should take care not to fall asleep; have a timer with an alarm at your side and set it for 20 minutes. A 500-watt heat lamp should be not closer than 30 inches. No matter what method of heat you use, the temperature should be comforting, not too hot. In addition, be sure to protect your arm from drafts and cold after the treatment. Heat can be used several times a day, and if you find it helpful, it may be continued for a week or more. If the pain is made worse, or if the heat is not helpful after three or four applications, it should be stopped. **A cautionary note:** Do not use heat if your arm and elbow feel inflamed, hot and swollen. Too much heat for too long a period can "cook" or burn the skin, causing permanent damage.

7. MASSAGE

This is a system of rubbing, kneading, stroking, pressing, or other similar techniques. It is one of the oldest methods used to relieve soreness and stiffness. However, your arm and elbow should not be massaged if they are severely inflamed, swollen, or painful when touched. Like heat treatment, massage is especially useful for mild cases of tennis elbow when there has been a strain and the arm muscles are sore and fatigued from too much activity. Massage is best done after a heat treatment. It can be done by a professional or by someone at home who is sympathetic to your problem and willing to do the massaging. (This could be a woman or a man; here, we have chosen a woman as our example.) The masseuse should be gentle and skillful, exercising great care not to irritate the tender area during the process.

To proceed: Place your arm, palm down, on a table covered with a pad, the masseuse facing you. She should apply dusting powder, baby oil, or rubbing alcohol to her hands or over your entire hand and arm in order to avoid pulling and stretching your skin. Then, placing her thumbs on top of your wrist with fingers underneath, she should stroke upward towards your elbow with gentle pressure. The pressure should be reduced near the elbow or most painful area and reapplied gently once this is passed, continuing up your arm to the muscles above your elbow. The descending touch should be light and caressing back to the hand-wrist area. The entire process should be repeated for five to ten minutes.

After the massage, don't expose your arm to cold air. Instead, wrap it in a warm towel or wear a warm sweater for protection. The process can be repeated twice a day, but it is essential that the massage be gentle and superficial, not deep and forceful. If it causes any additional pain, especially afterwards, the treatment should be discontinued.

These methods of home treatment are only part of the prescription for recovery. For best results, a special exercise program should be included with your rest and treatment. The therapeutic exercises, detailed in the "Exercises for Recovery" chapter, have been especially designed to avoid any additional pain and to speed recovery. They will improve the health and tone of the muscles, tendons, and ligaments usually involved in the tennis elbow syndrome. By conscientiously following these programs, you'll be able to return to the tennis court sooner and in better condition to play.

If your pain is in the 1 to 5 category, and if by resting your elbow for several days and perhaps following one of the methods of treatment in this chapter your pain has begun to subside, you should be starting the Exercises for Recovery. However, if your pain is severe, or persists, or worsens you must not hesitate to see a doctor.

FIVE
SEEING A DOCTOR

Unlike a toothache which sends you to the dentist, the early symptoms of tennis elbow are usually disregarded until the elbow is so painful that you can no longer continue playing the game. Three or four weeks, or even longer, may elapse before you decide to get medical attention. By that time your daily activities may also have become disrupted because of your inability to use your playing arm efficiently without producing pain.

Physicians throughout the world are becoming increasingly familiar with the mechanism and treatment of tennis elbow as the number of patients increases along with the growth and popularity of tennis. Usually, it is the orthopedist who is most familiar and helpful with tennis elbow, since he specializes in diseases and injuries of the bones, joints, muscles, tendons, ligaments, and bursas.

DIAGNOSIS AND SELECTION OF TREATMENT

The diagnosis of tennis elbow is fairly obvious with tennis players, since it is directly related to the activity of the game. To further evaluate the problem, the orthopedist obtains a medical history of the symptoms and sometimes requests selected laboratory tests and X-rays to eliminate the possibility of other pathologic involvements which may cause or contribute to the pain in the elbow. For example, the X-rays may indicate a previous fracture or a childhood deformity, resulting in faulty mechanics in the elbow; or, they may reveal calcium deposits, arthritis or a loose piece of cartilage, sometimes containing a fragment of bone. The laboratory tests may reveal high uric acid, in which case gout could be considered as a contributing cause of the elbow pain.

When all the evidence has been gathered, including a look at the patient's racket, his stroking technique, and his muscle development (especially of the forearm), an assessment is made to determine suitable treatment. The treatment is selected from the various methods available, depending on the nature of the injury, how long the patient has suffered with it, the intensity of the pain, and how it's affecting the patient physically and psychologically. The initial treatment usually includes a precise regimen of rest, medication, and specific therapeutic exercises.

REST

There is a variety of methods for resting the arm. The use of a sling was discussed in the "Home Treatment" chapter. However, many patients are not restricted enough by a sling and continue to extend and flex the wrist, causing further irritation to the damaged tissues in the epicondylar area. A doctor can ensure effective rest for the arm of such a patient by using a lightweight metal molded splint which supports the wrist in a slightly cocked position and lessens the strain on the forearm muscles. The splint should extend from slightly below the elbow to the knuckles in the palm, permitting comfortable use of the fingers; the base of the thumb should sustain no pressure, and the thumb should move freely. An elastic bandage, 2-to-2 1/2 inches wide, is suitable for holding the splint in place. The bandage should be loosely wrapped, especially around the wrist and between the thumb and index finger, so that it does not interfere with circulation. The splint may be worn to bed, and may be easily removed for washing and for therapeutic exercises such as those recommended in the "Exercises for Recovery" chapter. A sling may be used with the splint for additional arm rest and comfort.

There are some patients who require more complete rest and arm support than that offered by the splint. In this situation, a plaster cast would be used, extending from the armpit to the knuckles, with the elbow bent at 90 degrees. The cast would be open and easily removable for washing and the therapeutic exercises. This type of cast is more comfortably worn with a sling. A cravat sling is adequate. The muscles rapidly atrophy and lose strength if not exercised regularly, so a non-removable cast is not suitable for the tennis-elbow patient.

If relief is not obtained with cold or heat as previously discussed in "Home Treatment," the physician may suggest whirlpool baths, diathermy, or ultrasonic treatment. These methods should be used with caution, under the supervision of a registered physical therapist, and if a distinct improvement does not follow a few treatments, or if the pain is increased, the treatment should be discontinued.

MEDICATION

If aspirin, as discussed in "Home Treatment," combined with rest does not give adequate relief of agonizing pain, the physician may prescribe a narcotic such as codeine for a day or two. There are other medications that relieve pain and some of them also have an anti-inflammatory effect, but these drugs can have side effects with occasional serious complications. If these are prescribed, the directions should be followed precisely and if there is any adverse or questionable reaction, the drug should be stopped and the doctor notified.

A number of synthetic steroids in the cortisone family are available; they are very effective in reducing inflammation and relieving pain. Sometimes a pill in the cortisone family is prescribed, but only a minute fraction of what is ingested ever reaches the elbow, and there may be harmful systemic effects, especially if the drug is taken over a period of time; so oral cortisone is not recommended. A combination of cortisone and local anesthetic, skillfully injected at the site of the inflammation, is most effective and causes no systemic effects. The injection need not be very painful, and relief is promptly obtained in more than 90 percent of the patients. An immediate relief from the anesthetic, which lasts for two to three hours, confirms the accuracy of the injection. The cortisone effect does not fully develop for a day or two, so the pain may return in the interval, but it can be relieved with the use of a sling, cold application, and aspirin.

Cortisone is an anti-inflammatory agent with a prolonged effect that reduces tissue tension and pain. The relief should last for three or four weeks and may be permanent if the patient recognizes (and uses) the period of relief as an opportunity to allow the healing process to take place. Unfortunately, many patients are so elated with the immediate relief they receive from this treatment that they go back to the tennis court to misuse their arms in the same ways that caused the original injury. This treatment should not be repeated more than three times, especially at short intervals, since repeated injections of cortisone may cause tissue damage. It must be understood that the underlying causes of the pain are still there. The injection is not an inoculation against the recurrence of the pain, nor does it repair a lesion. The absence of pain should serve as an opportunity for starting a special arm exercise program to build muscle strength and restore health to the damaged tissue. (See "Exercises for Recovery," chapter 6.) In addition, this rehabilitation period is a good time for reviewing stroking techniques. (See "Correct Stroking," chapter 8.)

SURGERY

Although rarely used, surgery may be considered for severe and persistent tennis elbow which has not yielded to other kinds of treatment. Since the type of surgery varies with the nature of the injury and the source of the pain, we will not describe in detail the various surgical procedures. Briefly, the most common operation, and the simplest, concerns the tendon attachments to the lateral epicondyle, which may be divided, lengthened, or repaired by a plastic procedure.

Another type of surgery deals with the circular (annular) ligament of the elbow which, if it is damaged, may be divided, excised or repaired. Still other surgery is required to release a nerve entrapment, or to remove a piece of cartilage from the joint.

After any of these operations, the elbow is rested in a cast, wrist splint, or sling until the deep tissues heal, which may take several weeks. Usually, guided exercises are begun within a day or two after surgery to maintain joint and muscle function, and to promote good circulation, minimizing swelling, stiffness, and loss of strength. The exercises should be performed to favor, rather than interfere with, the recovery process. After all is completely healed, the exercise program should be gradually expanded to restore the elbow to full strength and activity, including conditioning for tennis.

SIX
EXERCISES FOR RECOVERY

Recently I saw a woman, thirty-five years old, with acute tennis elbow. She had been playing once or twice a week for the past three years. Recently she had acquired a beautiful, expensive new racket which she had been trying for several weeks. Unfortunately, she could never really play with it because of the increasing pain in her elbow, which became worse at each attempt. She had typical lateral epicondylitis with marked tenderness and pain on resisted motion.

I tested her forearm muscles and grip and found them weak. Then I asked her to demonstrate various strokes, using her new racket (which she had brought in at my request). She did them badly. I examined her racket: it was inflexible, tightly strung with nylon, and had a grip that was too large for her small hand. Is it any wonder she had tennis elbow?

I explained the possibilities and limitations of a steroid injection. She decided to try it, and so I injected the steroid into the tender area of her elbow. To her amazement, she had immediate relief. However, I was careful to explain to her that the injection was only part of the story. I suggested several corrections of her forehand and backhand strokes and asked her to do them for me. When she had them right, I told her to practice them after purchasing a different racket that was more suitable for her. She was to follow the exercises in this chapter, rest her arm in a sling part time, and use aspirin as prescribed. When she returned the next week, she told me that the pain had not recurred and that she was doing the exercises regularly. The exercises were increased, and she began racket-gripping and gentle shadow-stroking. After another week without pain, the exercises were again increased, and her strokes were again reviewed. Her form looked good. Finally she started playing, easy and not for long at first, but several times a week. She continued to make progress because she had done her exercises faithfully and had not tried to move ahead too fast.

Specific exercises (like the ones in this chapter) were the key to this patient's recovery, as they can be to yours. All are simple, easy to do and require no special equipment. They should be done regularly each day, preferably at specific times, or they can be done at odd moments if you are adequately disciplined.

Basically, rehabilitation of tennis elbow depends on a precise regimen of rest and exercise. Resting your injured forearm and elbow is important, but resting does not mean total immobilization or inactivity. Your muscles should be exercised regularly to maintain their vitality and tone. An unexercised muscle becomes flabby and unresponsive, then deteriorates. Our therapeutic program of rest and exercise is designed to prevent deterioration of the finger, wrist, forearm and shoulder muscles, to speed healing of the elbow, and to send you back to the tennis court as rapidly as possible.

Muscles constantly receive a certain blood supply, but this supply is small compared to that received when they are exercised. When you begin exercising, there is a great increase in the blood supply to your muscles, bringing oxygen and other nutrients to the area and carrying away waste products to be eliminated by your body. This speeds the healing process and makes your muscles firmer, more elastic, and more responsive. In addition, the specific exercises described here will nourish your elbow, promoting mobility and health by increasing its ability to produce and absorb the lubricating fluid that it normally manufactures.

The Exercises for Recovery have been arranged in progressive levels. Begin by reading through the exercises. This will help you determine what level in the program is appropriate for you, depending on the intensity of your pain and the mobility of your elbow. If your pain is moderate to severe, start in Level One and stay there as long as you find it necessary before proceeding to the next level.

The first rule in Exercises for Recovery is DO NOT INCUR PAIN. This means that your already painful elbow should not have additional pain either during or after the exercise. The second rule in Exercises for Recovery is TAKE IT EASY. You may be in a hurry to get well and proceed to the next level of the program, but if you do the exercises too quickly, jerkily, or forcefully, especially when you have pain, you may increase the pain and delay or prevent recovery. The third rule is EXERCISE REGULARLY. Try to do the exercises precisely as described. Do each day's exercise with the thought: "this is the day of recovery." Missing exercise days will delay the success of the program. Your objective is to eliminate the pain as rapidly as possible and restore the health of your elbow.

LEVEL ONE: Search and Find

This is a method of determining the best position for you to start exercising to receive the most benefit. Slowly and gently, bend your forearm across your chest, keeping it close to your body. (See diagram.) Keep your hand open and relaxed, palm facing your chest. Very slowly, open and close the fingers several times, making a fist; do not clench with power. If you feel pain, move your forearm up or down to another position and try again. Be patient; you may need to experiment to find the best position, that is, the one that does not increase the pain when you open and close your fingers. Your position may be with your hand directly under your chin, or at breast level, or slightly below, or at your waist. Once you have "found" the most comfortable pain-free position, you are ready to begin the exercise program.

In the "found" position, gently open and close your fingers 10 times, at least 10 times a day. This exercise takes only a few minutes and can be done while watching TV, sitting at your desk, waiting for a bus, waiting in your car for the light or for traffic, and at other odd moments. At the end of this exercise, straighten and bend your elbow as much as you can without causing discomfort. (If your pain is in the lateral epicondyle area, the most comfortable position is with your palm up. Turn your palm down if your pain is in the medial epicondyle area.) Don't straighten your elbow with force, and don't enter the pain zone. But don't hesitate to begin this exercise at once, even if it means straightening the elbow only very slightly each time. This action exercises the injured ligament. If the elbow is continuously immobilized, the injured ligament tends to shorten and, in time, this may result in restricted motion. Straighten the elbow to the point of no pain, and don't test it beyond that point. At this level straighten your elbow 4 or 5 times after each finger exercise. These two exercises should be done for at least three days before going on to the next level.

When you do move to the next level, do not rush through the exercises but observe how your elbow feels both during and after them. If you become aware of additional pain, you are not ready for Level Two, so return to Level One for two or three more days.

CAUTION: While recovering from tennis elbow, some players become generally inactive and so allow their physical fitness to deteriorate. Don't fall into this rut. Instead, use the time to improve your running endurance and do exercises that will strengthen your leg and stomach muscles. This will improve your performance on the tennis court when you resume playing. You might even do some exercises to improve the muscle tone of your other arm.

LEVEL TWO: Easy Does It

For the first week at this level, you should not venture out of the "found" position, except for straightening and bending

Search and find
the most
comfortable
position
to begin
the exercise
program

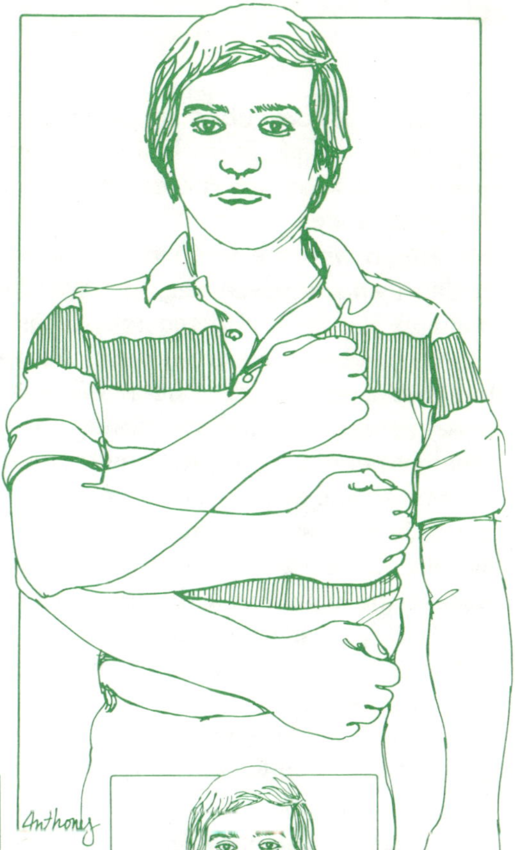

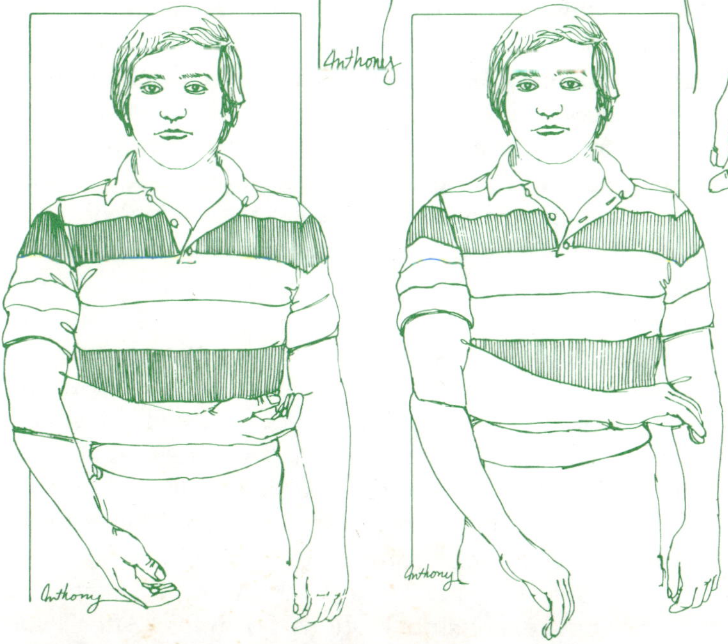

Straightening and bending the elbow gently is an important exercise for the injured ligament the elbow as described in Level One. For this exercise, a very soft synthetic foam ball is advisable. This type of ball is available at most toy stores; make sure it is soft and offers little resistance.

Begin with the foam ball in your hand at your "found" position and squeeze very gently. The squeeze should last about 5 seconds, and the release an additional 5 seconds. (Some people have a tendency to jerk their fingers open, but this is incorrect. The release is as important as the squeeze and should be done slowly and gently for the greatest benefit. You may time the squeeze-release by slowly counting until you get the tempo of it.) As you open your hand, feel your forearm muscles relax in the process. You should not feel any pain or discomfort while you squeeze or release the ball; if you do, try squeezing it more gently and slowly. If you still feel pain, you probably have not "found" your position and should return to Level One for the Search and Find exercise.

You may find the exercise more comfortable if you support your elbow with your other hand. **(A reminder: do not enter the pain zone at any time; if you do, you may perpetuate the injury.)** To proceed, squeeze and release the foam ball, as suggested, for 2 or 3 minutes as a test. Stop, rest, and feel. If you do not feel any additional pain, you can increase the exercise time to 5 minutes, at least six times a day. At the end of each squeeze-release exercise, do the elbow-straightening-and-bending exercise. As your elbow improves, straightening it will become easier; however, never force it in any way.

At the end of the first week, try changing the position of your squeezing hand. If your "found" position was high on your chest, drop it several inches; if your "found" position was at your waist, try a higher position. If you feel additional pain while performing the exercise outside of your "found" position, return to it and continue the exercise there until you can proceed without discomfort.

If you are able to squeeze and release at an alternate position, continue exercising in both positions. After two days, try the exercise in several positions up and down your chest.

REVIEW of Level One and Two Exercises

Your arm is flexed, across your chest, the elbow close to your body for support. Squeeze and release the ball slowly as described, never jerking your fingers open or closed. If you feel additional pain, do not do the exercise in an advanced position: instead, return to the comfortable one. Do the exercise for at least 5 minutes at a time, six times daily, but if you feel your finger or forearm muscles getting tired, take a break. Remember the straightening exercise after each squeezing exercise.

CAUTION: It is important at this level not to miss a day of the exercise program. You cannot make up for lost time by performing faster, or with more repetitions.

If you do miss a day or two, be especially careful when resuming the exercises, since your muscles may have lost some of their tone because of inactivity, and your elbow may be more sensitive.

LEVEL THREE: Getting Better

You are now at a stage in which your hand is in various positions when squeezing the foam ball. You're getting better! If you do not reinjure your elbow by misusing it or banging it, you will soon be making even greater progress.

It is now time to change from the foam ball to a rubber ball that has more resistance. A new or used tennis or paddle-tennis ball is ideal, depending on which you find most comfortable.

You are now very familiar with the squeezing and releasing method—do not change it except for using the rubber ball. Continue the squeezing and releasing exercise, always doing it slowly and deliberately and testing for any signs of pain. If you can squeeze and release the rubber ball with comfort for 3 to 5 minutes, you have come a long way from Level One and are now on the road to recovery.

Follow the next step carefully. You are going to try the

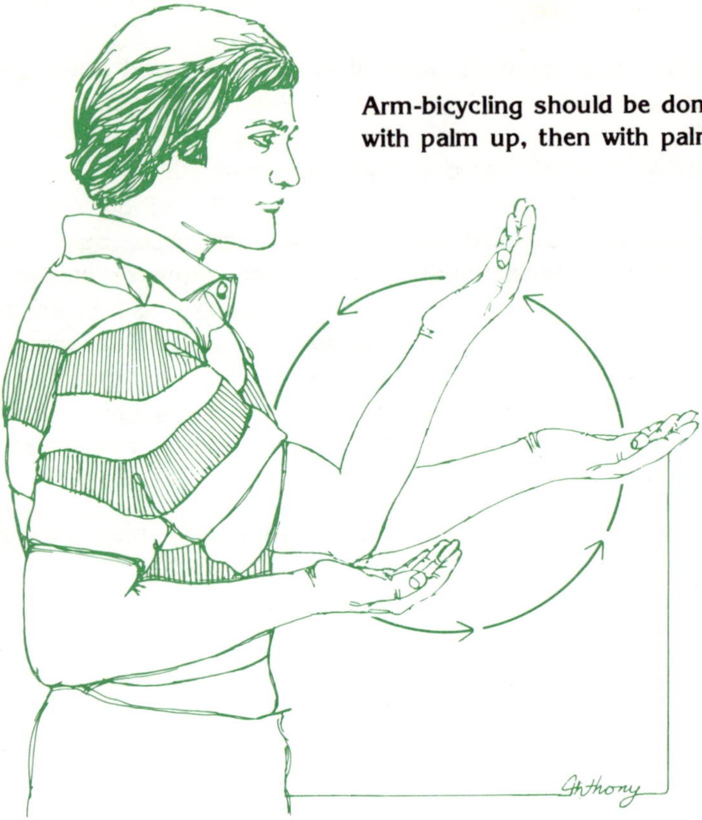

Arm-bicycling should be done with palm up, then with palm down

squeezing and releasing exercise with a partially extended forearm—like this: with rubber ball in hand, hold your elbow 4 to 5 inches in front of your body in a half-cocked position, forearm in front of you, and palm in mid-position, as in a handshake. In this position, test-squeeze and release the ball. You are now using the extensor muscles in your forearm to a greater degree, so be very careful—you want to determine if these muscles have healed sufficiently to perform the exercise without incurring pain. Try the test several times. If you are free of additional pain, continue this exercise with the elbow partially extended from your body.

For best results and to speed the healing process, this exercise should be done regularly, at least 3 to 5 minutes at a time, at least six times a day. You can stop for a short break if your fingers become tired or your muscles seem to fatigue; and then start again. At this point, you should notice a marked increase in the firmness of your forearm muscles—good insurance against recurrence of tennis elbow.

You have now progressed successfully in the squeezing exercise, so it is time to alter the elbow straightening-and-bending exercise in this way: with elbow bent and palm up, move your hand forward and then back toward the shoulder with a circular motion, like turning a bicycle wheel with your hand instead of your foot. This exercise is excellent for the elbow and shoulder joints and will increase the blood circulation in your entire arm; it should follow the squeezing of the rubber ball. Arm-bicycle with palm up at least 10 times, then 10 times with palm down. As you probably realize, these exercises can be done while you're on the telephone, watching TV, reading, or taking a coffee break. Be aware of those odd moments when you can do a few exercises, and take advantage of them. Keep an extra rubber ball with you in the car or in your handbag or pocket, and use it frequently.

CAUTION: If you are at this level, don't get overanxious and begin rushing the process. Continue gradually increasing the repetition of the two exercises, and you will soon be on the tennis court. However, if these new exercises cause any discomfort, you should return to Level Two until the healing process has progressed.

LEVEL FOUR: Dust Off the Racket

Does your racket meet your special requirements? Do you know whether it is head-heavy or if the grip is too large or too small for your hand? If you cannot answer these questions with confidence, turn to chapter 7, "Choosing the Right Equipment."

This next exercise should be done after you have squeezed the rubber ball and arm-bicycled. It is best done in front of a mirror, where you have sufficient room for a full backswing, stroke, and follow-through. Grip the racket firmly

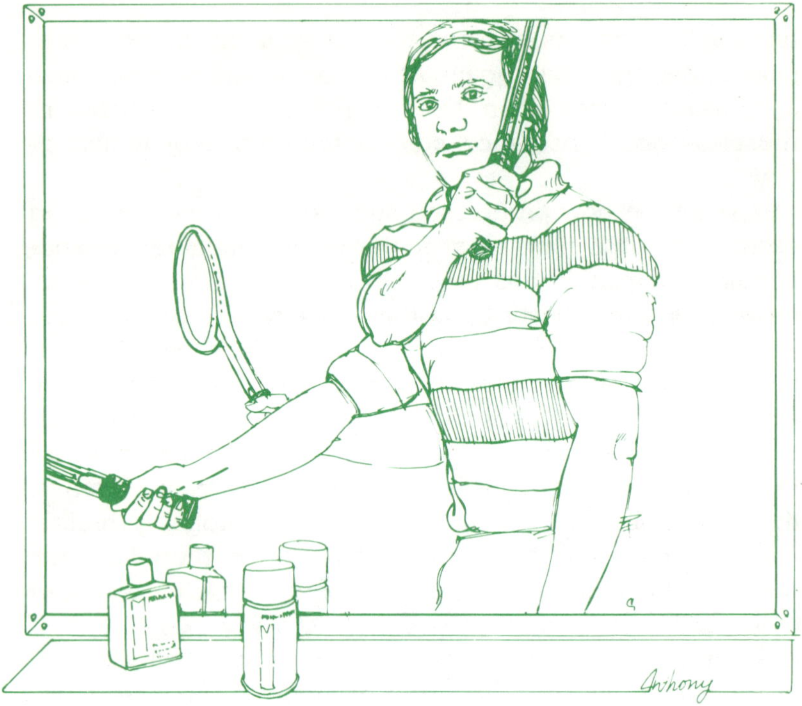

Forehand shadow-stroking in slow motion strengthens muscles

and support it at the throat with your left hand. How does it feel? If you have a slight forearm-elbow pain when gripping and holding the racket, you are not prepared for this exercise and should return to Level Three for a few more days or go through the stroking motions with your body and arm but without a racket.

Begin shadow-stroking with your forehand, trying for a very slow and graceful movement. This is not a contest, so don't attempt any of these strokes with power or speed. With speed, much that is incorrect is glossed over, and poor habits are formed. Watch your slow-motion movements in the mirror, or have a friend review your stroke, to make sure that the forehand is being done properly. Keep your elbow slightly bent throughout the backswing, stroke, and follow-through. This is an exercise for strengthening your muscles

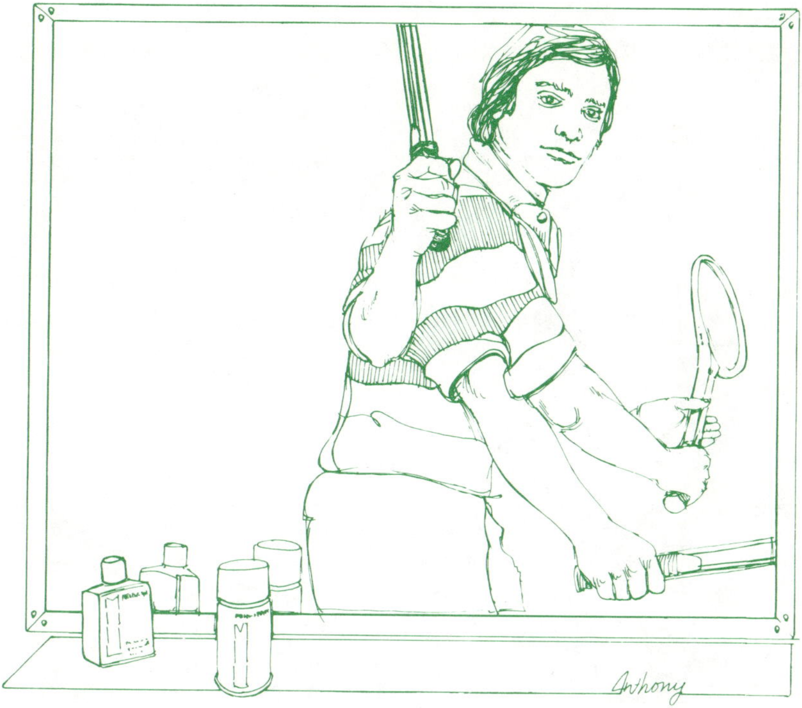

Backhand shadow-stroking in front of a mirror lets you observe and correct your stroking

and for making stroke adjustments and corrections. (See chapter 8, "Correct Stroking.")

You are still in therapy, so continue the Level Three ball squeezing, arm-bicycling exercises (at least six times daily) and forehand shadow-stroking (at least ten minutes daily). Take a break whenever you feel it necessary, and don't become fatigued. After several days, the forehand stroke should become comfortable and feel natural.

Before adding the backhand to your shadow-stroke exercises, read "Correct Stroking" (chapter 8) on the backhand. Then try a few backhand strokes, noting your form in the mirror. Remember that when you bring the racket forward to hit the imaginary ball, your weight should shift from your back to your front foot as you lean into the ball, the imaginary power coming from your shoulder as you hit

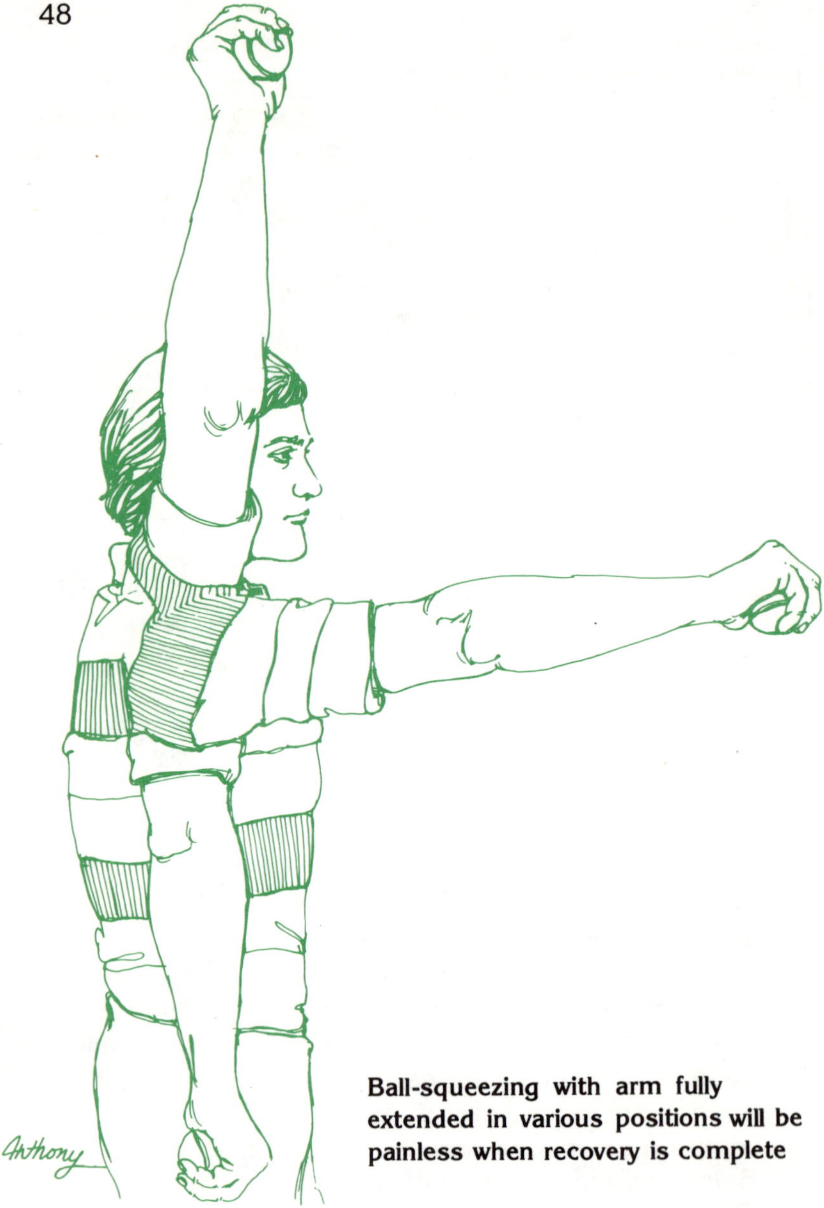

Ball-squeezing with arm fully extended in various positions will be painless when recovery is complete

and follow through. After a few backhand strokes, return to the forehand, alternating between the two as you develop your muscles and observe and correct your strokes. Always begin this exercise with a few minutes of forehand strokes before doing any backhand strokes.

There should be no pain during or after these stroking

exercises; if you are aware of any discomfort at your elbow, you are not yet ready for this or the final level.

LEVEL FIVE: Lace Up Your Tennis Shoes

If you have consistently followed the therapy program after entering the level that was appropriate for your elbow's condition, and stayed in each level until you were certain you should move to the next one, then the healing process should be complete. Your forearm muscles are now firmer, stronger, and more responsive.

The following is more of a test than an exercise: it will help you determine whether your elbow is completely healed, and if you are ready to return to the game.

Starting with your elbow in a half-cocked position, squeeze the ball as before for several minutes, slowly straightening your elbow so that your arm is fully extended in front of you. Can you squeeze the ball with a fully extended outstretched arm above your head and at your side? If you do not feel any pain when repeatedly squeezing the ball in these positions, you have successfully completed the Exercises for Recovery.

Read the next section, start the preventive exercise program and make your first post tennis-elbow date. Don't rush or overdo it; gradually start playing, increasing the time and frequency as you regain confidence in your elbow and reestablish your skills.

HOW TO PREVENT IT

Recognizing the many possible causes of tennis elbow and the methods of preventing it is essential if you wish to continue playing, free from the agony of the injury. If you have rehabilitated your elbow, you are not immune to recurrence unless you follow a program of prevention. If you have never had the problem, you are surely well acquainted with the casualties that occur on the courts and would prefer not to join that long list of dropouts. If you are a tennis instructor, your healthy elbow means your continued employment and continued personal pleasure in playing. The next several chapters will provide each of you with ready answers regarding the possible causes of aching elbows. In addition, if you are a teacher, they may serve as a handy reference as you guide your students in the correct principles and approach to playing better tennis.

SEVEN
CHOOSING THE RIGHT EQUIPMENT

THE RACKET

Among tennis players, the discussion goes on . . . "what is the best racket on the market?" You are faced with this dilemma when you enter any tennis shop and see wall-to-wall rackets. These rackets are produced and impressively advertised by a long list of consumer-oriented manufacturers, all hoping to convince you of the merits of their product. Our guidelines concerning racket choice relate to the prevention of tennis elbow. First of all, we dismiss the method of choosing a racket by the adage, "How does it feel?" Don't limit your judgment to "feel"; how the racket "feels" in the shop is quite different from the "feeling" during or after an hour of play. Your racket should fit your unique characteristics: the size of your hand, the condition and tone of your arm muscles, and the type of game that you now play.

Rackets are manufactured from wood, metal or composite (fiberglass or graphite). Within each category of material there are many variables to be considered when making your choice. Racket weight runs from a LIGHT 11 oz. to a HEAVY 15 oz. We recommend a LIGHT to LIGHT-MEDIUM weight, within the range of 11 to 13 1/2oz. A heavy racket causes muscle fatigue and will tire your arm and grip. It also causes a loss of stroke control and efficiency, leaving you more vulnerable to tennis elbow. Most tennis shops are equipped with scales so that you can make certain of the exact weight of a racket. Since quality rackets come without strings, the shop should provide a substitute weight that is attached to the head of the racket to compensate for the absence of strings when weighing it.

Do not purchase a pre-strung racket. Have your racket strung at a shop where they know their tennis business. A racket which is too tightly strung will send vibrations down the handle and into your arm. These repeated jarring vibrations are a factor contributing to tennis elbow. We recommend that your racket be strung at 55 pounds, except when the manufacturer of a particular racket specifies otherwise. If the range is 55 to 60 pounds, you should choose the lesser tension as a precautionary measure. Strings come in a range of nylon and gut qualities. A high-quality nylon is best suited for damp weather, since it will retain its tension. Gut loses its tension in damp weather and tightens when the weather is dry or cold.

The correct balance is of utmost importance in selecting your racket. Balance refers to the weight distribution of the entire frame. The head-heavy racket is particularly troublesome to the underdeveloped wrist and forearm. It can cause the wrist to sag, overstretching the forearm muscles, and this strain can lead to the onset of tennis elbow. All properly equipped tennis shops will test-balance a racket and advise you whether it is heavy, head-light or balanced. We recommend that your racket be level on the balance. If there is a slight dip towards the head (head-heavy), the racket should be rejected. We would approve a very slight dip towards the grip (head-light). If the racket is being balanced before stringing, a string-weight-compensator should be attached to the head, as in the weighing process.

Flex is another factor to be considered when selecting your racket. Flex refers to the bending of the racket from head to grip. Flexibility reduces racket vibration. A very stiff racket does not absorb the vibrations after impact but transfers the shock to your arm—once again, a possible cause of tennis elbow. The degree of racket flexibility is difficult for most buyers to determine, so it is best to rely on the advice of a competent salesperson at the tennis or pro shop.

The size of the grip, also called the handle, is of major importance in selecting your racket. An oversized grip will tire your hand, causing the racket to slip and turn on impact. An undersized grip will also tire your hand and may cramp the fingers as well. Grip sizes range from 4 to 5 inches in circumference and fractions in between. There is no exact formula for selecting the proper grip size because of the great variety of hand sizes. The method of finding the right grip that comes closest to a satisfactory answer is the one used by many racket shops: you shake hands with the handle. Then place the index finger of your free hand in the space between your fingertips and the heel portion of your thumb. If you cannot place your index finger in that space because your fingertips are too close to the thumb heel, then the grip is too small for your hand. If there is too much room for your index finger, most likely the grip is too large. Your index finger should fit snugly, but not tightly or loosely.

How to determine proper grip size

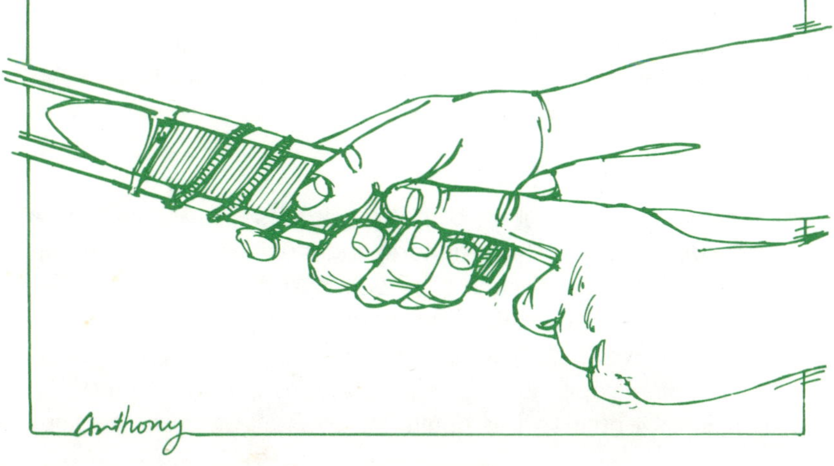

If your racket preference is wood, you should keep it in a press to prevent warping. An out-of-shape warped racket can be harmful to the health of your elbow. Such a racket will twist from head to grip on impact, overstretching and twisting wrist and forearm muscles. Also, it will exaggerate the vibrations on impact, causing further disturbance to your arm. If you already own a wood racket that has not been kept in a press, check it for warping. To do so, place the head of the racket on a flat surface; if the head wobbles or does not lie flat, do not play with it.

Many sports shops have a selection of demonstration rackets in all materials and sizes that are available for trial use. Since you can often try such a racket for several days, this is an excellent way of selecting one that meets your needs.

TENNIS SHOES

Shoes seem to be far removed from the site of the elbow, but the manner in which you get to the ball, and the position of your feet on impact, is related to the health of your elbow. (Footwork is detailed in "Correct Stroking," chapter 8.) The soles of your tennis shoes should have plenty of grip for rapid starts and quick stops. The soles of boating sneakers or worn-down tennis shoes cause slides and slips; and the inability to control your footwork causes you either to overreach, resulting in a stiff elbow on impact, or to get too close to the ball, resulting in a cramped elbow on impact. If either of these strokes is repeated over and over, you may be inviting tennis elbow.

TENNIS BALLS

For most locations it is best to purchase your balls in a pressurized can; for high-altitude locations the balls can be purchased in a cardboard box. You should buy high-quality balls because they retain their bounce longer. Balls that are worn and have lost their nap and bounce will interfere with your timing. Proper timing is necessary for correct stroking, which is essential to the health of your elbow and the success of your tennis game. Don't mix your used tennis balls with new ones; keep worn tennis balls together and use them for practicing serve and volley or hitting against a practice wall.

EIGHT
CORRECT STROKING

This chapter deals with methods of stroking, body and foot positions, and other techniques pertaining specifically to the problem of tennis elbow. It is not intended as a comprehensive guide to playing the game. You may wish to supplement our guidelines and improve your game generally by attending a tennis clinic or camp, taking private lessons, or reading the latest book by your favorite tennis star. And, if you can arrange it, have a friend take movies of you in action, including close-ups and slow-motion; then carefully analyze your strokes on film. In any case, before you practice these corrective strokes, it is essential that you warm up properly (detailed in "The Warm-Up," chapter 10).

YOUR GRIP

If you have never held a racket in your hand you will most likely acquire your grip technique from your first teacher. If you have played for several years and are not unhappy with your grip, don't attempt to alter it in a radical way. If you wish to make a change, do it gradually. A sudden major alteration will interfere with your stroke and might have dire consequences during a match. Your hand, wrist, and forearm muscles have become accustomed to your grip as well as your technique and will undergo strain when an alteration is attempted.

Do not clutch the handle of your racket tightly. Your grip should firm up when receiving the ball and relax after the impact and follow-through. When you temporarily stop playing during a match or practice to retrieve balls, change sides of the court, or simply rest, do not continue holding your racket with a firm grip; switch it to your other hand, or hold it lightly at the throat where it is in balance. These break periods are excellent opportunities for you to relax your arm, wrist, and fingers, allowing them to regain their vitality. If you continuously grasp your racket, you may tire or cramp your forearm muscles and cause an unrelenting tension in the epicondyle area.

Try to keep your racket handle dry during play by toweling the sweat off your hand and racket handle whenever possible. This is important because if your hand slips and you hit the ball slightly off-center, the handle may twist in your hand, causing severe strain to your forearm muscles. At a break in play, you may find it helpful to dust your hand and handle with resin powder, available in a small bag at any sporting goods store. In addition, when your racket handle covering begins to wear down, it will become increasingly difficult to keep it dry and grip it properly. When this starts to happen, get it re-covered at your tennis shop. In this case, a smooth finish is no help!

If your hands are sensitive and easily irritated, you can wear a special tennis glove designed for protection. Sore fingers and palms contribute to shifting and adjusting the grip; this in turn leads to poor stroking control which is, as we have mentioned, a major cause of possible damage to your elbow.

YOUR WRIST

Playing with a limp or weak wrist heads you on a one-way road to tennis elbow. A drooping wrist allows the racket head to drop below wrist level into a zone of no support on impact with the ball. It causes a sharp extension (forcing back) of the wrist joint on impact from a forehand, forehand

The grasped-wrist exercise corrects limp or drooping wrists

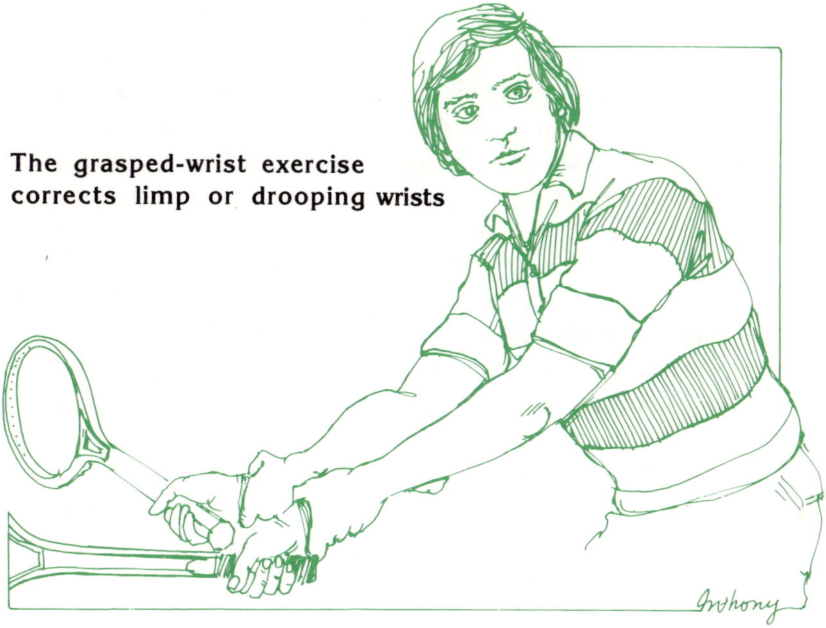

volley or return-of-service; and it causes an exaggerated flexion (forcing forward) of the wrist joint on a backhand, backhand volley or return-of-service. These repeated flexions and extensions of the wrist can result in damage to the groups of muscles in your hand, wrist, and forearm that lead to the elbow. A whipping wrist action can have similar damaging effects by making the direction of the racket head impossible to control. So be on the lookout for this, as well. When you hit the ball and follow through, your wrist should be firm and slightly cocked in a neutral position, supporting the head of the racket a little above wrist level.

You may not even be aware that you have a wrist problem, since it's difficult to discern its action during play. But, off the court, with racket only, you can conduct a simple test and repeat it as an exercise to correct your wrist problem if you find one.

Here's how: Get into position for your basic forehand stroke, with arm and racket back; now, grasp the wrist joint of your racket hand firmly with your free hand while you shadow stroke and follow through. Repeat this action several times. If you can feel your wrist joint moving under the pressure of your grip, you are stroking with wrist action. Test your backhand in the same way. To practice this "grasped wrist exercise," shadow stroke repeatedly 25 times with your forehand, then your backhand, several times a day. After a week or so, you'll find that your wrist is firmer and that you have better control of the direction of your racket head when you actually stroke the ball.

As we learned in our anatomy discussion (chapter 3), the mistake of following through with excessive wrist and forearm rotation on both the forehand and backhand is one of the major causes of tennis elbow. Repeated excessive pronation (palm downward) on the forehand or supination (palm upward) on the backhand causes exceptional trauma to the forearm muscles and their tendon attachments at the elbow. Therefore, it is most important to correct these stroking violations.

STIFF ELBOW

When you stroke with a stiff elbow, your racket is extended too far from your body at the moment of impact, and therefore you don't have the leverage you would get by stroking with your elbow slightly bent. Stroking with a stiff elbow is particularly distressing on the forehand because it forces the elbow joint back unnaturally, in the same way a door is forced back against its hinge, leading to possible ligament or bone damage at the elbow. In addition, stiff-elbow stroking is uncomfortable and tends to force the forearm to roll over on both the forehand and the backhand, resulting again in dangerous pronation and supination. When you are at the courts, observe the tennis player stroking with a stiff elbow. Note how awkward the strokes appear and how much energy is expended striving for power.

EYE-ON-THE-BALL

Watching the ball would seem to be the easiest and most obvious requirement of playing tennis. However, for most players at all levels, it is the most difficult and elusive discipline of the game. What exactly does watching the ball mean? It means continuously keeping your eye on the ball as it leaves your opponent's racket, flies across the net, (bounces), and contacts your racket. As you know, constantly watching the ball requires great concentration: you cannot allow yourself to be distracted by outside influences nor by your inner thoughts or emotions. If you cannot master watching the ball, your ability to get to it in time to execute an efficient stroke, and to make optimum ball-racket contact will be impaired.

You must take note of the ball as soon as it comes off your opponent's racket, or your start will be delayed and you will have to stretch to reach it with a stiff-elbow stroke; or you may misjudge where the ball will bounce, overrun it and be forced to use a cramped-elbow stroke. If you do not watch the ball as it bounces and hits your racket, you will hit it off-center, causing the racket to vibrate and twist in your hand. Repeated off-center hits will fatigue your hand, pain your forearm muscles and, ultimately, make your elbow sore.

All tennis players struggle to achieve concentration. Your awareness of this need will lead you to your own techniques of achieving it.

GET-THE-RACKET-BACK, GET-THE-RACKET-BACK

Tennis instructors repeat this reminder over and over for good reason. Getting your racket back early is essential, since you will stroke well only if you are prepared. How soon should your racket be taken back? As soon as the ball leaves your opponent's racket and you know whether it will be a forehand or a backhand: this is the answer most instructors will give. There should be no delay. Your racket should be taken back immediately, until it points to the fence behind you. This movement is also known as the backswing.

Here's a way of determining the correct timing of your backswing: As you move toward the ball, your racket should be brought back before you take your second step. If you follow this practice, you will be prepared to hit the ball out in front, and with power. If you delay taking your racket back, your stroke will be rushed and cramped and you will meet the ball late, resulting in a powerless stroke. You may attempt to compensate for this by relying on last-minute action from your wrist and forearm, thus increasing your elbow's vulnerability.

To protect your elbow, remember, too, that it should be slightly bent on the backswing and the stroke. This partial flexion relaxes your muscles, lessens the strain, and gives you more control and power.

Getting your racket back early requires awareness, concentration, and bushels of practice balls. It is one of the most important requisites for good tennis and a healthy arm.

THE FOLLOW-THROUGH

This is the natural course your racket follows after it has hit the ball. (The following indications are for right-handed players and should simply be reversed for "lefties.") For a correct follow-through on the forehand, your racket head, pointing in the direction you wish the ball to go, should continue to rise after it contacts the ball until it stops just above your left shoulder. The follow-through is similar for the backhand: the racket head stops high in front of you and slightly to the right of your right shoulder. (Some refer to this as the Statue-of-Liberty pose.)

Proper stroking and follow-through give direction and power to the flight of your ball. If you interrupt the follow-through by holding back, it is the same as pulling a punch—the ball has no power and, what's more, doesn't go where you want it to go. By stopping the natural flow of your follow-through, your racket collides with the ball instead of meeting it, and this collision transmits shocks to your forearm and elbow. When you follow through correctly, the forceful flow of your racket minimizes the impact of the ball and sends it in the direction you would like it to go.

Being aware of the position of your racket head as it stops at the completion of your follow-through is important in determining whether your forearm rotates excessively. If your racket head is rotated downward on completion of your forehand stroke, you have pronated your wrist and forearm; if it is rotated upward on completion of your backhand, you have supinated your forearm and wrist. As we mentioned earlier in this chapter, as well as in the anatomy discussion, this repeated forearm rotation is one of the major causes of tennis elbow. Watch for it!

THE BACKHAND

Running around the backhand is common among those who feel awkward and inefficient in performing it. The average player finds this stroke more difficult than the forehand to begin with, and it therefore evolves as his weak and defensive stroke. Tennis instructors and tennis books often state that the backhand should be easier to perform than the forehand because you swing away from your body instead of across it. While this may be true in theory, in practice the backhand remains a problem for most players.

Let's review the basics of the backhand stroke. (These indications are for right-handed players.) Starting from a ready position facing the net, you see the ball leave your opponent's racket, heading for your backhand; your left hand is at the throat of the racket guiding it back as your right hand switches to a backhand grip, and you pivot left by rotating your shoulders and torso. With your left hand still in place to stabilize and guide the racket, you move toward the ball, stepping forward with your right foot. As you step, you shift your weight from the (left) back foot to the (right) front, uncoiling your body and leaning into the stroke. You contact the ball in front of your right foot and follow through naturally, as described before.

If the backhand stroke is not executed correctly, it can

be the most uncoordinated and least reliable stroke of the game. And, no doubt about it, the backhand position and stroke seem alien to many beginning and intermediate players. There may be a good reason for this attitude: the backhand stance and stroke are different from any other action that we perform. For instance, most of us can comfortably swing a bat or a golf club in a manner similar to the forehand, so that the movement is not awkward (though it may not be correct). But if we try to swing from the opposite shoulder, as in the backhand, we swing awkwardly and without grace. This is because we are unaccustomed to this type of action and have had little experience with it. As a result, the extensor muscles which perform the backhand are less developed than the flexors involved in the forehand.

The poorly coordinated backhand overloads the extensor muscles: for instance, if you fail to shift your weight from the back to the front foot when stroking, your forearm extensor muscles receive the full impact of the oncoming ball transmitted from the racket. As mentioned earlier, the strain travels up the extensors to their tendon attachments at the lateral epicondyle where the damage takes place. This is further complicated if the hit is off-center and the forearm is supinated on the follow-through. (The supinator muscles also attach in the lateral epicondyle area of your elbow.) Therefore, correcting an improper backhand stroke is of major importance in the prevention of tennis elbow. If your backhand stroke is troublesome, you should have it analyzed by an instructor who will suggest how you can correct it. With attention and practice you can improve the elements of your stroke and achieve the necessary timing, power, and control. Some players favor the two-handed backhand for protection as well as for added power.

TOPSPIN, SERVE, VOLLEY

Topspin is **not** achieved by rotating your wrist and forearm so that the racket head rolls over the top of the ball. As already discussed, this rolling action is potentially harmful to your elbow. Topspin is achieved by stroking forward from a low to a high position and maintaining a vertical racket head throughout the stroke.

The serve requires a series of coordinated movements: the backswing, so-called back scratch, ball toss, weight shift, hit, and follow-through. As contact is made with the tossed ball, the arm is fully extended and the wrist snap requires the muscles in the forearm to stretch from an already taut position. To condition these muscles for the strain of serving, a long warm-up is essential. As a further precaution, forehand and backhand strokes should be practiced before attempting serves; and prolonged service drills should be avoided by interspersing them with other practice strokes.

The forehand and backhand volley are most often executed at the net and are used more frequently in doubles. When you are at net, you are receiving the ball at close range and therefore with greater speed. Concentration, a constant eye-on-the-ball, fast reaction, and a ready racket are prerequisites to a successful volley.

To ready yourself for a volley, hold the racket well out in front of you with the top of the racket head about nose level. At no time should you bring the racket back—always keep it prepared in front of you. The volley is a short punch-like movement with some shoulder and elbow action. If you allow the racket head to drop too low, or if you bring the racket back, the chance of hitting weakly and off-center is greatly increased. Off-center hits at net can be especially jarring to your arm and elbow because of the high velocity of the ball.

One special note of caution: Opthalmologists are reporting an alarming increase of eye injuries sustained by being hit in the eye with a fast-flying ball at net. If you do come to net often, or if you play doubles, you should wear special protective eyeglasses designed to prevent this serious injury.

Finally, playing when fatigued is a cause of out-of-control strokes, slow reactions, late starts, overreaching, wrist-forearm whipping and other actions that can cause pain to your elbow. Although we have described many of these faults in detail, you must remember that repeated poor stroking of any kind can lead to elbow problems; and you are more liable to stroke poorly when you are tired. So, do not play to the point of exhaustion—call for a break or call it a day—your game, your elbow, and your entire body will be the better for it.

NINE
PREVENTIVE CONDITIONING

GENERAL HEALTH

The tissues, muscles, and bones of the body, its glands, circulatory and digestive systems and organs, are all closely related. If you neglect one part of your body, other areas usually become adversely affected. Therefore, the maintenance of general good health is important in the prevention of tennis elbow.

Your overall physical fitness is something you become aware of immediately when playing tennis. Can you move to the ball with agility? Are your muscles strong enough for the power you need? How good is your coordination, your endurance? There are no shortcuts to acquiring these components of physical fitness. They depend on sufficient hours of rest and sleep, proper diet, a regular program of exercise, and the elimination of excess weight, smoking, excessive drinking, and the use of harmful drugs.

Books abound dealing with easy exercise programs, miracle diets, and the elimination of tension. They tell you how to look younger, feel better, and live a longer and happier life. Many of these fast-diet, speedy shape-up books are of little value, since there is no quick and easy road to good health. However, there are books available that offer sound nutritional advice and a reasonable approach to the development of physical fitness. We suggest you look for these to supplement our guidelines in establishing your program of total physical fitness.

If you are an adult and have no regular exercise program, are fifteen pounds or more over your healthy weight, smoke a pack or two a day and feel generally tired even before tennis, you don't have to be told that you are in poor physical condition. It is essential that you have a medical examination before starting any exercise program or continuing to play tennis. After age 60, or even 50 if you smoke, drink, or are overweight, a stress electro-cardiogram evaluated by a cardiologist competent in this test would be desirable. Doctors generally don't prohibit exercise but may limit the intensity and duration of it until you are better prepared for vigorous activity.

Who is most vulnerable to tennis elbow? Weekend players. Saturday-Sunday wonders who sit at a desk or drive a car from house to work, to supermarket, to bridge, to school or PTA five days a week, then rush out on weekends (or on a two-week vacation) to give their all on the tennis court. Unfortunately, these players are more vulnerable, not only to tennis elbow, but to a constellation of other injuries sustained on the courts. And, tennis is not the only culprit; injuries result from general activities such as lifting, carrying, snow-shoveling, or gardening. As an orthopedist, I see several weekend "athletes" each day. Then, too, there's the former athlete who comes in on Monday morning, crippled after three or four sets of tennis on Sunday. "I must be getting old," is the usual refrain. These people forget that, in earlier years, they spent hours training and conditioning every day.

The intelligent athlete-tennis player prepares for the game in four ways:

1. Conditioning the whole body
2. Conditioning for tennis
3. Warming-up thoroughly
4. Practicing the correct strokes

Weekenders often skip these preparations and go directly to play. But, there is no need to be a weekend athlete even though you only have time for tennis on Saturday and Sunday. During the week you can do exercises that suit your physical condition and your personality. Select exercises that don't bore you or require more time than you can give regularly. Your purpose is to improve your strength and endurance and to prevent tennis elbow as well as other injuries.

Tennis is a stop-and-go-sport, with frequent moments of rapid activity, requiring sudden surges of heart, lung, and muscle action. Sustained rallies, long sets and matches require endurance and reserves of stamina. As we have said, exhaustion leads to a loss of coordination, stroking control, and concentration. When you are tired, you may whip your wrist and arm, and you will tend to mis-hit the ball. Any of these factors can lead to tennis elbow. So don't be a weak weekender!

WHOLE-BODY EXERCISES

To improve endurance, there is no better exercise than jogging or running. An excellent lung-heart-circulation conditioner, it also strengthens muscles, lubricates joints, and induces a sense of well-being. Tennis players who run a mile or two, five or six days a week, have little difficulty sustaining their endurance during a tennis match. Like all vigorous exercises, however, running should be developed gradually, increasing distance and speed by degrees. You may start by walking, then walk-run-walk, and so on. (In some cases, depending on physical condition, brisk walking only should precede running for the first few days or weeks.)

Running is the best of the whole-body exercises since it requires no special equipment and can be done almost anywhere, in almost any weather, in a minimum of time. Other suitable endurance-building exercises are walking vigorously for several miles, swimming, rope jumping, rowing, and bicycling, although the latter is primarily for strengthening the leg muscles. In order to benefit from any of these exercises, you should do them regularly: before breakfast, or two or more hours after a meal, at least four times a week.

A word about breathing, which so many of us take for granted because its a natural life-sustaining function: people have a tendency to hold their breath when exercising. Holding your breath, even momentarily, while playing tennis or exercising should be avoided since it interrupts the oxygen supply, thereby decreasing your energy and depleting your strength. Become aware of your breathing when you are playing tennis; practice breathing deeply when drill stroking or exercising. When you breathe deeply and rhythmically, you won't tire as easily, your strokes will be more natural, and your game will improve.

SPOT EXERCISES

There are many types of exercise that, applied to specific muscles, will condition them and make you less prone to a tennis-elbow injury. For instance, isometrics, a system of tensing one set of muscles against another, increases muscle tone, although it does not move the joints or promote circulation. Isometric exercises are especially useful when you don't have room for movement, such as at a desk, in a car, or some other confined space. Then there are stretching exercises which gradually lengthen tight muscles, warm up muscle areas, and relieve tension; and exercises against resistance, such as weights and springs—again, excellent for toning and building strength. The most desirable exercises cause the muscles to contract and relax rhythmically, rather than be held in prolonged stretch or contraction.

Before you begin any of the spot exercises for the prevention of tennis elbow, take a few minutes to warm up your body. Run in place, stretch your arms and legs, and do a few calisthenics. The warm-up will slowly increase your heartbeat and your body temperature. Each time you warm up before an exercise, you will avoid stiff and aching muscles the morning after. Don't force an exercise or hurry through it. Exercise with coordination and precision, allowing yourself sufficient time to perform at an easy pace, without exhausting yourself or reducing your capacity for the next day. The exercises should be done progressively, that is, increasing the number of repetitions as they become easier. "Warming down" toward the end of the exercise period will also help to prevent stiff, sore muscles.

These physical exercises will help you achieve and maintain physical fitness in the muscles of your hand, wrist, forearm, upper arm, and shoulder so that they can withstand the rigors of playing tennis. However, these exercises, alone, will not prepare you completely. Select a couple from each category and plan a program around a combination of these and swimming, running, or rope jumping. Incidentally, swimming, rowing or using a punching bag are particularly good exercises for strengthening the generally weak extensor muscles. Set aside a specific exercise time, at least four or five days a week. Don't forget, it's regularity that's important.

WARNING! You should not attempt any of the following exercises if you have tennis elbow. Your elbow should be fully recovered and free of pain before you start.

Push-Ups

Push-ups are excellent for arm-shoulder muscle development. If you cannot do a full push-up from the floor, start with a half push-up, supporting your weight with your hands and knees instead of your feet. Or, start with your hands at the edge of a table, dresser, or windowsill—with body straight and arms extended, alternately bend and straighten elbows. Another type of push-up is done sitting in a chair that has arms strong enough to support your weight. With

Half push-up promotes arm-shoulder development

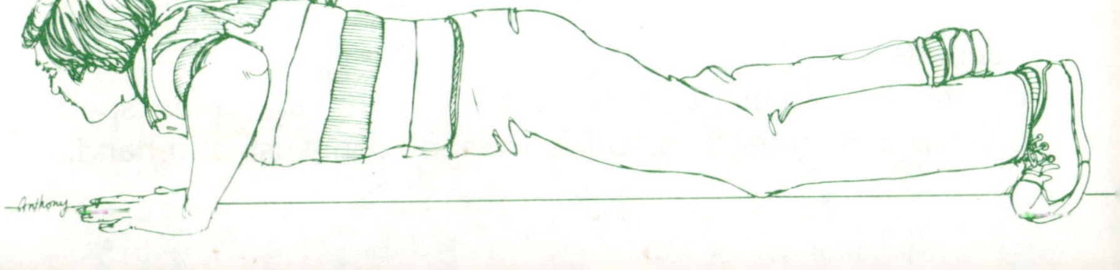

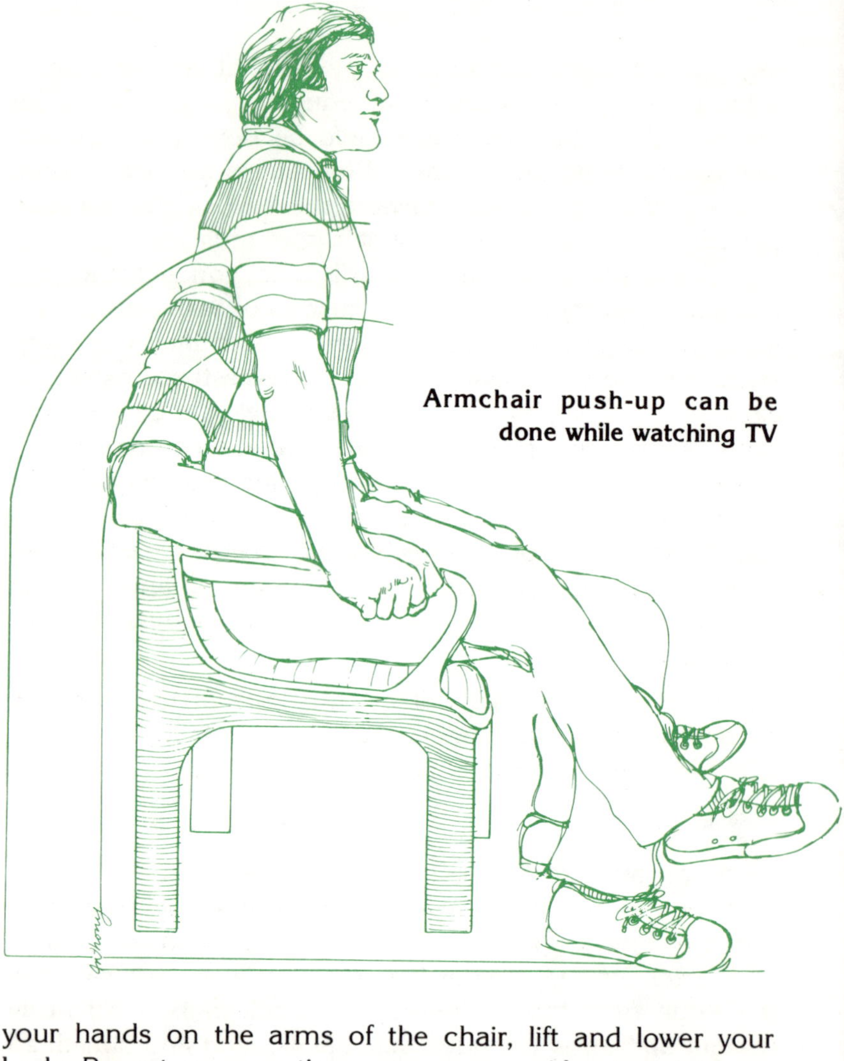

Armchair push-up can be done while watching TV

your hands on the arms of the chair, lift and lower your body. Repeat as many times as you can without straining or fatiguing your muscles. After a week of modified push-ups, once again try a full push-up; it will seem easier than before. Chin-ups and other arm bar work are also good conditioning for tennis.

Dumbells

Dumbbells or hand weights, properly used, can rapidly spot develop and strengthen your arm, shoulder, wrist, and hand.

The usual starting weight of "bells" is from 3 to 5 pounds each for women, and from 5 to 10 pounds each for men. (These ranges are broad; the right weight for you depends on your physical condition.)

Prepare an exercise chart to keep a record of your progress. Record the exercise, the day, the number of repetitions, and the dumbbell weight. Don't attempt to rush the program; instead, stay with the number of repetitions that you can do with ease before increasing them. In any case, stay at each repetition level for a week, and don't increase the number of repetitions by more than two or three in any one week. For best results, do the exercises slowly and evenly without strain, breathing deeply as you do them.

Exercises for Shoulder and Upper Arm

1. Stand with feet about 12 inches apart, holding a bell in each hand at shoulder level, elbows bent. With your right arm push bell slowly upward until arm is fully extended overhead, then lower bell back to shoulder level. Repeat with left arm, alternating back and forth, 5 to 10 times for each.

2. Stand with feet about 12 inches apart, holding a bell in each hand. Raise bells to shoulder level, then stretch arms out to the side as far as they can go, palms facing forward. Now, slowly rotate arms, making 3 small circles to the front. Then repeat, making 3 small circles to the rear. Repeat exercise 3 to 10 times.

3. Lie on floor, holding bells at shoulder. Extend right arm upward until it is fully extended, then lower bell back to shoulder. Repeat with left arm, alternating back and forth, 5 to 10 times for each.

4. Stand with feet together, holding bells with an undergrip lowered at your sides. With your right arm, curl the bell to your shoulder, and lower it to your side. Repeat with left arm, alternating back and forth, 5 to 10 times for each.

5. Sit erect in a chair, palms up under a heavy desk or table, forearm level with the top surface, elbows comfortably

bent. Push up, hold the count to 10, relax, repeat 5 times. Breathe deeply while counting.

Exercises for Wrist and Forearm

1. Sit in a chair, rest your right forearm on your thigh, your wrist extended beyond your knee. Hold the bell in the right hand, palm up. Allow your wrist to extend slowly toward the floor, lowering the bell as far as it will go comfortably, then curl your wrist upward as far as possible. Your forearm should not move but remain supported on your thigh. Repeat 5 times and then 5 times with your left hand, or do the exercise with both wrists together.

2. Assume the same position as in Exercise 1 (above), except that the bell is grasped with an overgrip, palm down. Repeat the exercise in the same way as Exercise 1, with the same number of repetitions for each hand. Perform both exercises slowly, allowing only the wrist joint to move the bell up and down.

For Exercises 3 and 4 you may require a lesser weight than in the previous exercises, since the muscles used may

Isometric exercise to strengthen forearm muscles by pressing up with right forearm and down with left hand (see exercises 4,5, and 6 opposite)

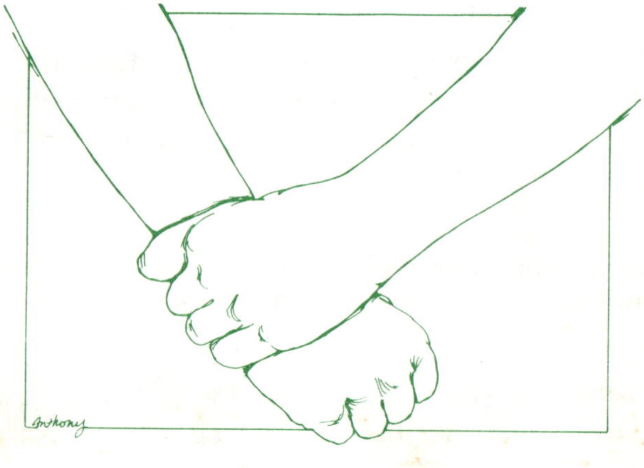

not be as well developed. You might try a book or a rock or a full soda can if you don't have smaller weights.

3. Assume position as in Exercise 1. Hold bell in right hand, palm up, and pronate counter-clockwise while your forearm remains resting on your thigh. Supinate back to the starting position so that your palm is up. The rotation should not be done with abrupt action, but with precision and control. Repeat 5 times, then repeat with left hand.

4. In a standing or sitting position, extend arms in front of you with elbows slightly bent, palms up. Grasp your right wrist firmly with your left hand and press up with your right forearm and down with your left hand, holding the tension for a count of 10. Stop and relax. Repeat 5 times for each forearm.

5. Repeat Exercise 4 grasping your palm.

6. Repeat Exercises 4 and 5 with your palm down.

Exercises for the Grip

Developing a strong grip is essential for preventing tennis elbow and improving your performance as a tennis player. You can strengthen your grip by squeezing a ball or a spring squeezer, available at most sporting goods stores. Alternately, you can squeeze a roll of sponge rubber or a sheet of newspaper shaped into a tightly wadded ball, or you can squeeze your opposite wrist. Whatever you use for squeezing, it should fit your hand well and be firm enough to use day after day and really exercise the grip. If you can squeeze the device fifty times, it is too soft, and your effort is being wasted.

Squeezing a device incorrectly is not only wasted effort but can cause pain in your hand and forearm muscles. To prevent this, your elbow should be bent about 90° when you begin the squeezing exercise. Squeeze slowly to a slow count of 5, then release to a slow count of 5. Many people tend to jerk open their hands on the release, thereby greatly reducing the effectiveness of the exercise. After squeezing and releasing 10 times in the bent elbow position you can extend your arm and continue the exercise. These exercises are not being done properly if they cause pain or discomfort while you're doing them, or afterwards. Repeat the squeezing and releasing exercises at least several times a day, or more often if you like. The exercises can be done while you are on the phone, in your car, at a desk, watching TV, or whenever you have a free minute or two.

A weak grip can be strengthened in a relatively short period of time if the exercises are done regularly and according to the directions given. I have had patients who, through diligent exercise, were able to double their strength in three or four months, as measured on the grip meter.

If you faithfully follow a routine program of spot and whole-body exercise, your general physical condition will improve greatly, as will your performance on the court and subsequent enjoyment of the game. If, in addition, you now have the proper equipment and have corrected your strokes, you are well prepared to play healthy and effective tennis. But, to reduce further your chances of getting tennis elbow, even while adding speed and power to your game, you must never forget the final step in conditioning: the warm-up.

TEN
THE WARM-UP

In 1965, there were about five million tennis players in the United States. By 1976, that figure had leaped to between thirty-five and forty million. To say that tennis is enjoying an unprecedented popularity growth is an understatement—tennis is having a popularity explosion; it is booming. Despite the fact that thousands of new courts are being constructed each year, playing time remains at a premium on both public and club courts.

Municipal courts are so crowded that even though local communities generally enforce an hour's limit on playing time, it is difficult to schedule the hour. Because of the crush, many private clubs have been forced to limit their members to doubles only on weekends; and commercial court fees have skyrocketed from a few dollars an hour to $25.00 or more in some areas.

These overcrowded, time-limited conditions are not conducive to what was, until recently, a customary ten minutes or more of warm-up on court. That period of leisurely preparedness has all but disappeared. Today, the ball generally crosses the net only a few times before one of the players yells, "Ready? Let's play"; and the game is on, full speed. Unfortunately, this precipitous rush into the vigorous action of the game, without an adequate warm-up, is a major cause of a variety of injuries to the ligaments, tendons, and muscles. Of course, some players race through the warm-up because it delays "the real fun" of the game, that is, a chance to win. Do not be overwhelmed by a need to score immediately, for this attitude can easily lead to weeks of no score and no fun at all.

There is no way to avoid it: warming-up is essential. Power and speed applied to cold muscles and tendons can tear them, especially around the shoulder and elbow where the load of action in tennis takes place. Warming-up energizes your entire body: you breathe more deeply, your heartbeat increases, and circulation becomes more active; there is a rush of blood and oxygen to your muscles and tendons so that they become warmer, more elastic, and better prepared for the vigorous extensions and contractions they will undergo. In addition, warming-up mobilizes the joint fluids, making the joints more flexible and easier to move.

Besides preparing your body to undertake the action of the game, the warm-up on court provides an opportunity for you to begin concentrating and focusing your eyes on the ball. (You have already learned how important this is for the prevention of tennis elbow in "Correct Stroking.") It allows you to become acquainted with the surface of the court, how the ball bounces on it, how the wind is blowing, and how this affects the flight of the ball. It gives you time to size up the technique and skill of your opponent. The warm-up accustoms you to the entire environment of the court—how your eyes react to the background or to the action on the courts nearby—so that when your game starts, these elements will not surprise or distract you.

Consider the warm-up a period of grace: a time to breathe deeply and clear the mind of anxieties, thus relaxing tense muscles; a valuable time that should not be wasted by merely ambling onto the court and getting your equipment out of your bag. Your racket and tennis balls should be ready for use. You should be wearing a lightweight sweater or jacket in warm weather, or a sweatsuit in cold weather.

Begin the warm-up slowly, stroking smoothly and precisely, always keeping your eye on the ball when it is in play.

At first don't try to hit hard or return difficult wide balls. The warm-up should be a gradual process of increasing the power of your strokes and the tempo of your foot movements. If you have had a problem with tennis elbow, hit only forehand strokes for five minutes, even if it means running around your backhand for that time. As you begin to warm up and develop a light sweat, remove your suit or sweater and continue to speed up the pace of your movements. As your body warms and your muscles become more supple, you can go for the more difficult balls as well as to the net for a series of practice volleys and overhead smashes. After your volleys, return to the baseline for additional ground strokes, both forehand and backhand. As you reach the final stages of the warm-up, and only then, start hitting serves from both the deuce and ad courts. As mentioned in "Correct Stroking," during the serve your arm is fully extended and some wrist snap is required on impact, making your muscles and tendons most vulnerable to strain. If your arm has been sufficiently limbered and warmed, that vulnerability is greatly reduced.

If, because of time or money, you prefer not to use the court for an extended warm-up, then it is important to warm up before getting on. Running, bicycling, or even vigorous walking for a mile or more to the court is an excellent way to warm the leg muscles and to start lung and heart action in preparation for the game. If you must use your automobile to get to the court, use whatever waiting time there is for traffic or lights to exercise your playing arm by squeezing a ball or other squeezing device; and bicycle your arm to loosen the elbow and shoulder joints.

No matter how you get to the tennis court, try to arrive at least a half hour before you are to play. Instead of sitting on a bench waiting for the court to become available, start your warm-up like any professional athlete. Remember to keep your body warm with clothing until the pace of the game has developed sufficiently to sustain your body warmth. You can begin with these simple limbering-up exercises that will warm and stretch your muscles:

1. Forward Trunk Bend. Standing erect, reach your fingertips toward your toes. Start slowly, breathing deeply and rhythmically, flexing your knees slightly if necessary. (Forcing with knees straight may strain the lower back.) Return to the erect position, repeating the bend 10 times.

2. Half-Knee Bend. Standing erect with feet about 15 inches apart, arms extended forward, keeping your heels on the ground, bend knees halfway. Return slowly to the erect position, repeating the half squat 10 times. If you are limber and strong, do this exercise with a full knee bend.

3. Run in the vicinity of the tennis court, or in one place if you must reserve your position for the court. Remember to breathe deeply. You can, if you like, squeeze a ball while you are running. Be careful not to exhaust yourself before the game. If you become tired, stop, and do an easier exercise.

4. Windmill. Start with arms extended out to the side at shoulder level with elbows straight. Swing arms slowly down, across your chest, up over your head, and out to complete the circle. Synchronize your deep breathing. Repeat the movement 20 times, then reverse the windmill action and repeat 20 times.

5. Shadow-Stroking. This exercise is excellent for the final phase of your off-court warm-up. You can go through the positions and movements of all the strokes with racket only and an imaginary ball. You can control your pace, speeding up and slowing down at will.

Beginning with the forehand shadow-stroke, move with correct footwork to a spot where the imaginary ball is to bounce; pivot, rotating your shoulders and torso as you take the racket back; then step forward, shifting your weight from your back foot to the front, as you make contact with the imaginary ball. Your elbow should be slightly flexed as you hit and follow through, being careful not to rotate your wrist or forearm. After you have executed a dozen or more strokes in different positions with your forehand, alternate it

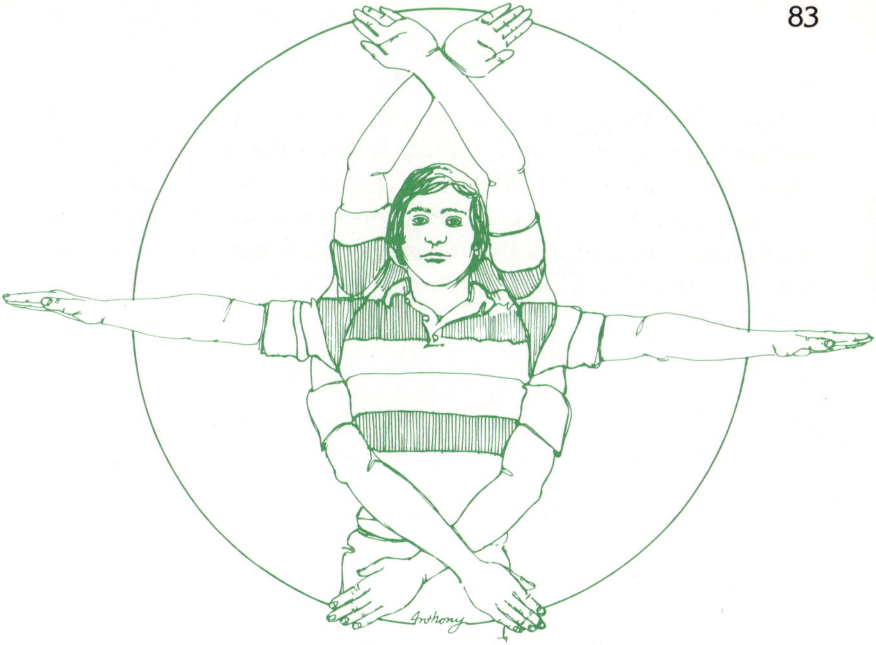

Windmill exercise is ideal for warming up

with your backhand, always concentrating on the imaginary ball and performing the basic actions fundamental to each stroke.

Practice the shadow-serve last; begin with a gentle stroke, not trying to overpower the imaginary ball. Take your racket through the service movement, paying attention to your grip, stance, back scratch, and follow-through. As you continue the serve exercise, you can exert more power, until your racket creates a swooshing sound as it goes through the air. Be careful not to overdo it in effort or repetitions because, as you have learned, the very nature of the serve places an extra strain on your muscles, particularly if they are underdeveloped or if you stroke incorrectly.

The primary objective of the warm-up is to prepare you physically and psychologically for the game. Tennis is fast-moving, requiring agility, flexibility, stamina and muscle power. When you neglect the warm-up, you are taking unnecessary risks and reducing your potential efficiency as a player. Of course, there's a chance of accident in most competitive sports, and tennis is no exception. You will, however, reduce that risk and prevent many aches and pains if you adhere to a common-sense warm-up period. The added dividend is that you may be spared the discomfort and disability of tennis elbow.

FINALS

ELEVEN
FADS AND FANCIES

We live in an age of instant solutions to a wide range of problems that once required time and effort to resolve. Advertisements on television and in other media keep reminding us that food preparation no longer requires time and energy, what with prepackaged dinners, frozen pancakes, waffles and pizzas, instant soup, tea, and coffee readily available in the supermarket. New developments in communication and computerization provide instant news coverage, cameras that develop photographs in 30 seconds, and the promise of one-minute loans and instant banking. There are remedies that claim fast relief for headaches, indigestion, constipation, and insomnia. Courses in speed reading are available for those who wish to read a book in an hour. Planes can fly you to Paris in time for lunch.

The Electronic Jet Age has generated the concept that the "immediate" is good and can be expected in every area. This push-button attitude is so pervasive in modern society that it has penetrated our ideas concerning health and our "right" to fast cures. Medical advances in the past fifty years—"miracle" drugs and inoculations—have, in fact, contributed to our expectations.

Many tennis players with the early symptoms of tennis elbow refuse to acknowledge it and continue the process of injury until the pain is so severe that they can no longer grip the tennis racket. Then, having sought help, these patients often expect immediate relief from pain with no disruption of their tennis-playing activities. When they are told of the proper medical treatment, the need for stroke correction and gradual development of their physical condition, they look upon this advice as coming from the Dark Ages. What they do expect is a "miracle" drug for instantaneous and permanent relief, and the assurance that tomorrow's tennis appointment will not have to be cancelled.

Even when the pathology of the tennis elbow injury is discussed with them in detail, many patients are reluctant to follow a program of recovery and prevention. The failure of an "instant" correction leads a large group of tennis-elbow victims to reach out for a variety of exotic and quick cures that are usually worthless. Not only do some of these devices and techniques offer no relief from tennis elbow, but many cause additional damage when the patient, relying on the magical cure, abandons medical advice and continues abusing his elbow. With this in mind, let's examine some of the popular "cures" and relief agents and discuss the myths and merits, if any, of each.

COPPER BRACELETS

Copper is one of the first metals known to man; it was probably mined several thousand years before Christ. Early man attributed mystical powers to the important resources in his world and copper ranked high in ancient times. Since then it has been used for tools, coins, and ornaments.

Copper bracelets, plain and ornate, costing from $2.50 to $100.00 and more, persist as the most popular device used by athletes to "cure" them of pains in the hand and arm. They are also worn as amulets to ward off the possibility of any future pain or disability. In the late 1800's, copper pennies were worn in the shoe to prevent rheumatism; in the 1940's the penny moved to a slit in the popular loafer as decoration.

The fad of the copper bracelet has caught on with many people suffering from arthritis. Arthritis pains often come and go, and when they temporarily go, the wearer attributes the relief to the bracelet, believing that somehow it promotes healing: by "trace-action," some copper penetrating the skin, entering the bloodstream, and altering the acidity of the body, or as an "electrical force."

More often the wearer will proclaim, "I don't know how it works, or if it works, but it can't do any harm."

The Arthritis Foundation has done research and has analyzed the effects of copper on and in the body and has found no causal relationship between copper and any cure or pain relief. In spite of these findings, the fad of the copper bracelet thrives and has been adopted by some tennis players to cure or prevent tennis elbow. If the copper bracelet reminds you not to rotate your wrist or forearm while stroking the ball or acts as a prompter to correct other techniques that can cause tennis elbow or aggravate the condition, then, of course, it does have value. However, any such jewelry or a simple piece of string worn around the wrist could be as effective.

ACUPUNCTURE

Acupuncture, which originated in China, is an ancient art of healing that involves the insertion of needles into various parts of the body to relieve pain and cure illness. The practice is based on the theory that certain points in the body are directly related to the internal organs and that these organs can be affected by rotating the inserted needles at the acupuncture points.

In the late 1960's, sensational reports of the painless wonders of acupuncture burst upon the Western world. Its anesthetic and curative powers were hailed and soon many untrained people were setting up practice as acupuncturists. It has since become clear that acupuncture is no painless panacea. Today, among licensed physicians, there are differing opinions as to its effectiveness. According to some acupuncture experts, it can sometimes give temporary relief of pain and may be useful in cases where Western medicine has little else to offer. However, other doctors think that whatever continuing effects it may have are due to psychological suggestion and conditioning—the placebo effect.

Regarding the application of acupuncture to tennis elbow: a great deal of reliable scientific investigation is still required if it is to replace or supplement any of the traditional procedures which, when properly administered, have been found to be effective. Basically, acupuncture has no direct effect on what's wrong inside your elbow, although in some people it may be followed by a psychological diminution of symptoms.

BANDS AND BRACES

As one observes the tennis courts of the world, another phenomenon appears: a strap-like bandage wrapped around the upper forearms of many players. To anyone unfamiliar with the game, this band might be considered a part of the tennis uniform. Its widespread use is further evidence of the extent of the tennis-elbow problem among players.

The most familiar of the forearm bands is a 2-to-3 inch rubber-cotton band with an adjustable velcro strap that applies pressure on the upper forearm just below the elbow. The more sophisticated of these bands contains a hard rubber pad that can be adjusted to apply direct pressure to the painful area of the forearm muscle. These arm braces are sold at most sporting goods stores and pro shops, as well as through mail order companies that advertise in many of the tennis magazines. Generally, the companies do not make specific claims for the product, other than: "it helps support weakened muscles," or, "it eases elbow pain." The pressure exerted by the support band on the forearm partially immobilizes the muscle, limiting the jerks on the tendons attached to the epicondyles. In addition, the band supposedly absorbs some of the damaging vibrations which, transmitted from racket to elbow, could further aggravate the tennis-elbow injury.

Another brace, less familiar than the pressure band, is a sleeve-like, semi-rigid appliance that is laced around the forearm and lower half of the upper arm. This device maintains the elbow in a half-cocked position, allowing it only a few degrees of motion when the racket is swung. The slightly bent elbow reduces tension on the extensor muscles and on the tendons in the affected epicondyle area. The tightly-laced brace also inhibits forearm rotation on forehand and backhand strokes, thus preventing further damage to the pronator and supinator muscles.

For those of you not troubled by tennis elbow, never wear a band or a brace as a preventive measure while playing. Both devices inhibit the full functioning of the arm muscles and prevent proper strength development. If you have tennis-elbow symptoms and are compelled to use a band or a brace to reduce pain while playing, consider it a temporary measure only. Don't let it become a crutch or a substitute for the complete rehabilitation of your elbow through therapeutic exercise and correction of stroke techniques. In addition, never wear either type of device when not playing tennis; by compressing the arm they reduce blood circulation and interfere with muscle action in the very area that requires these functions for healing.

THE "PLAY IT OUT" MYTH

Some stoics and some who have never experienced the severe pain of tennis elbow advise continued playing, even though the forearm muscles and the elbow may be sore. They mistakenly believe that the muscles, having endured enough pain, will suddenly learn their lesson and somehow return to good health. Unfortunately, this type of thinking can lead to increased injury and complications, greater inflammation of the injured area, and prolongation of the recovery period.

BEWARE!

Don't be enticed by potions, herbs, and electric healing machines, some of which are sold through the mail as miraculous pain killers. Don't rely on faith healing, laying on of hands, manipulation, or "bloodless" surgery. In a phrase: beware of all claims for instant sure cures for tennis elbow; there are none!

TWELVE
IT'S UP TO YOU

We hope that we have cleared whatever misunderstandings you may have had regarding tennis elbow. As you are probably now aware, there is no mystery to the injury. If you have it, you can cure it and prevent its recurrence. If you don't have it, you can avoid getting it. Of course, the chance of accident and the vulnerability of the human body are facts of the active sports life. But being well prepared minimizes the possibility of injury.

In tennis, as you have learned, being well prepared consists of a combination of factors. If the racket you now play with is not right for you, buy one that is suitable and have it properly strung. Essential, also, are correct stroking techniques, footwork, and body movements. These can be improved through instruction and practice drills. If you are new to the game you can begin with good habits and good technique. If you have been playing with bad habits, don't be discouraged, they can be corrected. Persist, and you will soon find these skills becoming easier. And remember, be kind to your body and your elbow. Always warm up.

Staying physically fit is another link in the chain of preparedness. It doesn't require expensive equipment or prolonged instruction. All you need is a suitable exercise program and your commitment to it. When you follow a plan of exercise for physical fitness over the years, it is your assurance of a long and zestful life both on the tennis court—and off. You may follow the remarkable example of May Sutton Bundy who won at Wimbledon in 1905 and in 1907, and then returned there as a quarter-finalist thirty-four years after her first major title. At the age of 85 she was playing great tennis—and winning.

It's up to you!